First published in 2024 by **Lotus Publishing**, Apple Tree Cottage, Inlands Road, Nutbourne, Chichester, PO18 8RJ, and

Human Kinetics, 1607 N. Market Street, Champaign, Illinois 61820

United States and International
Website: **US.HumanKinetics.com**
Email: info@hkusa.com
Phone: 1-800-747-4457

Canada
Website: **Canada.HumanKinetics.com**
Email: info@hkcanada.com

Illustrations and Photographs **Sanni Sorma**
Art Direction and Design **Sanni Sorma**
Printed and Bound **Replika Press Pvt Ltd., India**

Medical Disclaimer
This publication is written and published to provide accurate and authoritative information relevant to the subject matter presented. It is published and sold with the understanding that the author and publishers are not engaged in rendering legal, medical, or other professional services by reason of their authorship or publication of this work. If medical or other expert assistance is required, the services of a competent professional person should be sought.

British Library Cataloging-in-Publication Data
A CIP record for this book is available from the British Library

Library of Congress Cataloging-in-Publication Data

Names: Steele, Paul, 1954-author. | Brandelius, Angelica, other. | Glemme, Anders, other.
Title: Yin yoga 50+ / Paul Steele ; Contributors Dr. Angelica Brandelius, MD. PhD., Anders Glemme, Lic. physiotherapist.
Other titles: Yin yoga fifty+
Description: First edition. | Nutbourne, Chichester ; Champaign, Illinois : Lotus Publishing, Human Kinetics, [2024]
Identifiers: LCCN 2023017081 (print) | LCCN 2023017082 (ebook) | ISBN 9781718227071 (paperback) | ISBN 9781718227088 (epub) | ISBN 9781718227095 (pdf)
Subjects: LCSH: Yin yoga. | Stress (Psychology) | Joints--Range of motion. | BISAC: HEALTH & FITNESS / Yoga | HEALTH & FITNESS / Exercise / Stretching
Classification: LCC RA781.73 .S74 2023 (print) | LCC RA781.73 (ebook) | DDC 613.7/046--dc23/eng/20230501
LC record available at https://lccn.loc.gov/2023017081
LC ebook record available at https://lccn.loc.gov/2023017082

ISBN: 978-1-7182-2707-1
10 9 8 7 6 5 4 3 2 1

YIN YOGA 50+

SLOW FLOWS TO RESTORE YOUR BODY, IMPROVE FLEXIBILITY, AND RELIEVE PAIN

PAUL STEELE

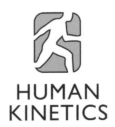

HUMAN KINETICS

FOREWORD

The movement of the human body can help improve your health and your experience of life in different ways.

Physical exercise can contribute to resistance against illnesses as well as relieving existing illnesses and diseases. For example, physical training can lead to a healthier cardiovascular and immune system, better blood sugar regulation, and stronger bone structure. Your brain is influenced positively by physical exercise through better mood and a greater ability to learn and concentrate.

Your mind and body are dynamically integrated and constantly influence each other. Through movement and breathing you send signals inward affecting your thoughts. And the other way around—your thoughts strongly influence your physical condition.

Yoga in different forms includes strength training, mobility, neuromuscular training, recovery, and mental training. In yin yoga, focus is on static stretches and practicing mindfulness.

Mindfulness—or conscious presence—focuses on the present through your senses and breathing without evaluating your experience. By directing attention inward, you can be more conscious about how you feel, what you think and how you are, leading to a greater understanding of yourself. Training your attention on what to focus may increase your ability to concentrate in everyday life.

Involuntary physiological processes including blood pressure, heart rate, digestion, and respiration are regulated by the autonomic nervous system. Parts of the autonomic system—the sympathetic and the parasympathetic systems—influence stress levels in the body. They cooperate and are always active to a different extent. The sympathetic system prepares you for fight or flight by the release of adrenaline, noradrenaline, and cortisol. This makes your heart rate, blood pressure, and respiratory rate increase. On the other hand, the parasympathetic system directs processes in your body to recover, heal, and helps you to rest and digest. Your heart rate, blood pressure, and respiratory rate slow down. Favoring the parasympathetic system, yin yoga may work as a powerful tool to recover from the effects of stress.

The different yin yoga positions, very well described in this book, may improve your range of motion, and work to prevent illness and enhance performance.

If you have not tried yin yoga before, you will find this book a great introduction, presenting many of the poses. For the more experienced reader, you will find this book a good reference and inspiration to new flows.

Enjoy.

Dr Angelica Brandelius MD, PhD

DR ANGELICA BRANDELIUS

MD PhD
Dr Angelica Brandelius is a personal and medical trainer (The Academy, Sweden) and yoga instructor (HiYoga Flow Foundation Teacher Training Course, 80H).

Angelica is especially interested in how physical activity in different forms can function as a powerful tool to achieve better health and performance in the different phases of our lives.

She leads classes in yin yoga/yoga, running, cycling, and strength training.

ANDERS GLEMME

Licensed physiotherapist
Anders Glemme specializes in preventing and treating sports injuries and offers orthopedic therapy for patients with movement issues in their spine, joints, discs, ligaments, and muscles.

Anders also has experience in rehab training, fascia treatment, Kinesio Taping, acupuncture and medical laser therapy. Anders has been a registered physiotherapist for over thirty years.

Contents

1

Introduction
AGE IS JUST A NUMBER

The point of this book is to help people "of an age" to live as full a life as possible and to offset the effects aging has on our bodies—and even our minds—by practicing yin yoga.

Your chronological age doesn't have to be your biological age. We all know that by avoiding smoking, not drinking too much alcohol, eating lots of vegetables, and getting the right exercise, helps.

But maybe we need more? And maybe yin yoga is what provides that "more"?

YIN YOGA IS NOT ALL CHANTING AND INCENSE

Many people have the wrong idea about yoga. They think it's all about trying to sit in impossible poses, making strange chanting noises, lighting candles, and quietly whispering "Namaste" to everyone around them. If you want to do any of these things, that's fine, but yin yoga is all about improving your flexibility, boosting your circulation, and reducing tension.

PERFECT FOR PAIN RELIEF

Lots of fifty+ people I talk to tell the same story. They wake up in the morning feeling stiff, and sometimes in pain. We all know why. As we age, our muscles become tighter and our joints stiffer. Part of the reason is that the body produces less synovial fluid that lubricates our joints. The other is reason simple.

We don't stretch.

Yoga helps us relieve pain in our joints, stretch our muscles and connective tissues, and even increase the production of synovial fluid. That means less pain, more freedom and a better life. Other research shows it even strengthens your bones [1].

YIN YOGA BENEFITS
EVERY BODY...AND MIND

The deep breathing exercises in yin yoga help reduce stress, lower your blood pressure and increase your immune defenses, all things that help you get a good night's sleep[2].

In other words, there are lots of physical, mental, and emotional benefits you gain from regularly practicing yin yoga. This book will hopefully give you the tools and the inspiration you need to start to practice this soft, slow yoga form.

And best of all? You don't need to be a super flexible person to do it. Everyone benefits from yin yoga, regardless of your physical and mental condition when you start.

I hope you enjoy the book and look forward to feeling even better – and younger.

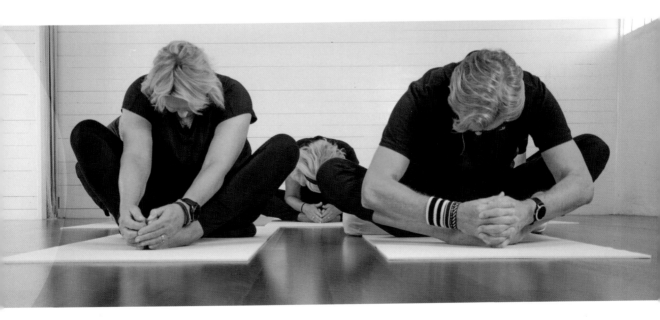

(1) https://europepmc.org/article/pmc/pmc4851231

(2) https://www.health.harvard.edu/mind-and-mood/relaxation-techniques-breath-control-helps-quell-errant-stress-response

WHAT IS
yin yoga?

Yin yoga is a more passive form of yoga that's good for our minds as well as our bodies. It gives us greater range of motion while lowering our blood pressure, giving us a greater feeling of well-being.

When we practice yin yoga, we use passive, longer held stretches or poses that allow us to get deeper into our bodies. We target our connective tissues – ligaments, joints, bones, and the fascia. The result is improved flexibility, better circulation, and less tension.

Yin yoga is nothing new. It's just a Western take on ideas about yoga and meditation that have been around for thousands of years.

WHY YOU SHOULD PRACTICE YIN YOGA

There are so many benefits to yin yoga for people over 50, from improving your mobility to lowering your blood pressure. Here are some of the major reasons you should practice yin yoga often.

Fixes issues with your tissues

As we get older, our joints and connective tissues tend to fuse together. This can be from repetitive jobs, from sports, or even from sitting for long periods. Often this causes pain and limits your mobility. The gentle stretching of yin yoga strengthens your connective tissues, reducing pain and inflammation. It's particularly good for conditions like arthritis.

Makes you more flexible and restores your range of motion

By holding poses for a longer time in yin yoga you can promote a deep release of your connective tissues, encouraging them to stretch. This helps increase your range of motion, meaning things like cutting your toenails or sitting on your heels become possible once again – after many years of neglect.

Gives you a flashier fascia

Fascia is connective tissue that holds every organ, blood vessel, bone, nerve fiber, and muscle in place. It's designed to stretch as you move but tightens up if you're stressed or you haven't used your muscles and joints. The result can be painful.

When we hold longer yin yoga poses, we promote elasticity and resilience in our fascia that could be lost through inactivity, strengthening our joints and increasing range of motion. That makes it easier to pick that golf ball out of the hole or swing your hips while doing that stylish carving turn when you're skiing.

Reduces stress and anxiety

Yin stimulates your parasympathetic nervous system, the rest-and-digest system. It reduces your heart rate, relaxes your muscles, and lowers your blood pressure.

Lets your body and mind become calm and still

Deep breathing, relaxation, and holding a yin yoga pose for a longer time means you relieve the stresses and strains of everyday life. It's a great way to remember your body and forget your to-do list, helping you reach new levels of rest and renewal.

Gives you an acupressure massage

Stretching and compressing your tissues stimulates the meridian lines. According to Traditional Chinese Medicine (TCM), these are the channels that enable our energy or "Qi" to run through our bodies. The theory is that this helps increase energy flows and restores balance in our bodies and minds. A large amount of research, such as that documented by the National Center for Complementary and Integrative Health[1] into acupuncture and acupressure shows that these practices do our bodies a lot of good.

Improves Your Memory

According to The Harvard Medical School[2], yoga helps improve memory better than brain training. Apparently, yin yoga and other yoga styles positively impact the brain parts responsible for processing information and memory. As yin yoga relieves stress, it also helps the brain to function more clearly.

Helps You Sleep

As we age, we become light sleepers. This can increase the risk of depression. The focus on meditation in yin yoga helps you sleep better by increasing melatonin [3] which is responsible for helping us sleep. Also, the associated breathing exercises help us relax – and sleep better.

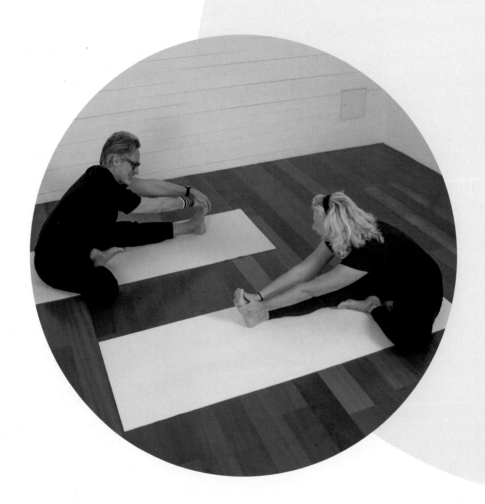

Boosts your sex life

Yep. It's true. Even for people our age. According to a study in the Journal of Sexual Medicine[4], yoga, and to some extent yin yoga, improves sexual function, particularly in women over 45. After 12 weeks of yoga, women participating in the study showed improvements in desire, arousal, lubrication, orgasm, and satisfaction. It's believed that yoga poses (asanas) improve core abdominal muscles, aid digestion, strengthen the pelvic floor, and lighten your mood.

Another idea is that yin yoga poses stimulate the kidney meridian (more about meridians below), helping remove blockages that may be holding you back from optimal sexual health.

There's some evidence it's good for erectile dysfunction[5] too, even if you're undergoing radiotherapy for prostate cancer. Patients who did yoga twice a week during a course of radiation therapy saw a significant reduction in sexual dysfunction as well as improvements in urinary incontinence and fatigue, compared with those who didn't do yoga.

So. Hit the mat for a friskier life after fifty!

SOME THINGS TO THINK ABOUT

As someone who discovered yin yoga a bit later, I see no drawbacks. But there are some things we ought to think about before we start practicing. A good idea is of course to consult your doctor before you start.

Be careful if you…

…have osteoporosis

As we get older our bones can deteriorate, leading to osteoporosis. In the United States alone, over 53 million[6] people have low bone mass and could suffer from the disease. If you suffer from osteoporosis, you should be careful when performing postures with spinal flexion (forward bending). These include Butterfly, Reclining Twists, Caterpillar, Saddle, and others. The stock answer is of course to see your doctor before embarking on a yin yoga journey.

The level of stress on your body—anyone's body—should be not too little and not too much. In his book, *Your Body, Your Yoga,* Bernie Clark, probably the most prolific yin yoga author, talks about what he calls the "Goldilocks philosophy." As he points out, too little stress leads to atrophy, fragility, or degeneration/shrinkage of muscle or nerve tissue. Too much stress can lead to serious damage. However, Bernie Clark feels that just the right amount of stress can lead to antifragility.

The actual point of stress that is right for you is called "finding your edge," which we talk about below.

...just had surgery

If you've just had a knee/hip replacement, you need to take things easy. But yin yoga is a great way to improve flexibility as you get better.

Yin yoga is probably an excellent complement to your physiotherapy as it stimulates the connective tissues around the replaced joint.

...have serious health problems like a heart condition

Again, consult your doctor, but yin yoga is a perfect way to improve your basic health by reducing respiration and heart rates, improving insulin sensitivity, normalizing cortisol, lowering stress, and thereby lowering your blood pressure. Go for it.

(1)   https://www.nccih.nih.gov/health/acupuncture-what-you-need-to-know

(2)   https://www.health.harvard.edu/staying-healthy/yoga-for-better-mental-health

(3)   https://www.ncbi.nlm.nih.gov/pmc/articles/PMC3328970/

(4)   https://www.medicalnewstoday.com/articles/323003

(5)   https://www.verywellhealth.com/yoga-for-erectile-dysfunction-poses-benefits-risks-5200227

(6)   https://health.gov/healthypeople/about/workgroups/osteoporosis-workgroup

3

A BRIEF HISTORY
of yin yoga

Yin yoga is one of the newer forms of yoga that started in the 80s by people experimenting with long-held stretches to see the effects on their flexibility. The founders of yin yoga say its inspiration comes from ancient Chinese Taoist practices of stretching and meditation.

That explains why yin yoga both targets the physical aspects of stretching while including elements of Traditional Chinese Medicine.

YIN YOGA AND TRADITIONAL CHINESE MEDICINE (TCM)

TCM has been used in China for thousands of years. What makes it different from Western medicine is that TCM uses a holistic approach that looks at your entire mental and physical well-being, and not just at treating a specific disease or ailment (normally with a drug).

Qi, the life force and the basis of TCM

According to TCM, Qi or Chi (think Qigong, Tai Chi) is a life force, energy that runs through everything, including our physical bodies. Practitioners believe that when your Qi is out of balance, you suffer both mentally and physically.
One way to put back that balance and improve the flow of Qi is yin yoga.

Proponents of TCM believe that yin yoga helps improve energy flows, letting Qi flow better to your organs, curing all types of conditions, from reducing pain to enhancing your mood.

YIN AND YANG–OPPOSITES THAT MAKE YOU WHOLE

Almost everyone recognizes the yin and yang symbol – the opposites that TCM practitioners believe are interconnected and must be in balance for our bodies to be in harmony by enabling Qi to flow unhindered.

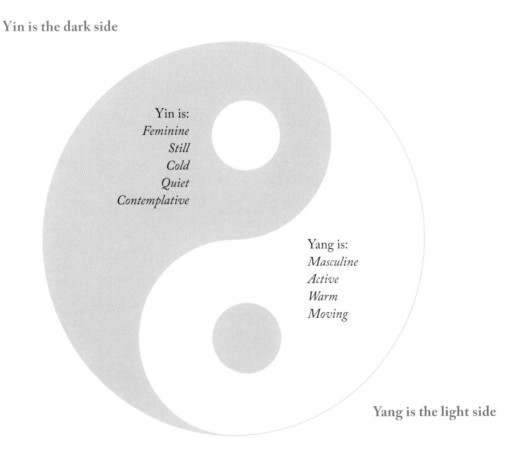

Yin is the dark side

Yin is:
Feminine
Still
Cold
Quiet
Contemplative

Yang is:
Masculine
Active
Warm
Moving

Yang is the light side

MERIDIAN LINES—
CHANNELING ENERGY THROUGH YOUR BODY

TCM talks about pathways called "meridians" that send Qi and energy through our bodies, and moisten our connective tissues (joints, tendons, fascia). If these channels are blocked for any reason, then the body doesn't function properly. Think about when blood gets blocked, or oxygen can't be absorbed.

In TCM there are 12 main meridians and several minor ones. The main meridians are connected to an organ. There are six yin and six yang meridians, each balancing the other.

The yin meridians are Heart, Spleen, Lung, Kidney, Pericardium, and Liver.

The yang meridians are Small Intestine, Stomach, Large Intestine, Bladder, Triple Energizer, and Gallbladder.

Because we need yin and yang for balance, most of these meridians are paired.

The Stomach meridian (yang) flows to the Spleen meridian (yin)

The Gallbladder meridian (yang) flows to the Liver meridian (yin)

The Bladder meridian (yang) flows to the Kidney meridian (yin)

The Heart meridian (yin) flows to the Small Intestine meridian (yang)

The Pericardium meridian (yin) flows to Triple Energizer meridian (yang)

The Lung meridian (yin) flows to the Large Intestine meridian (yang)

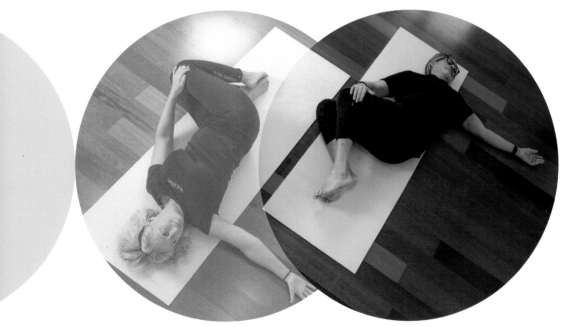

MERIDIAN LINES AND YIN YOGA

Yin yoga is based on creating conditions to open the meridian lines and let energy flow. By stressing or compressing our connective tissues, we are also stressing our organs, and in turn releasing any blockages in our meridians. As most yin yoga poses affect the lower body, then we mainly stimulate the Stomach/Spleen, Liver/Gallbladder, and Kidney/Bladder meridians.

Meridian	Physical benefit	Mental/emotional benefit
Kidney	Filtering waste from the blood and nourishing the marrow, the source of our red and white blood cells. In TCM, the Kidney meridian includes the adrenal glands, responsible for fight-or-flight reactions, as well as supporting sexual and reproductive functions.	A balanced kidney helps us feel safe and secure, gives us energy, enthusiasm, and drive. It also balances fear. If we have lower back problems, it's often a cause of blockage in the Kidney meridian, and means we feel fear, which causes tension.
Bladder	This meridian runs through the back of the heart, activating the parasympathetic nervous system, inducing relaxation. When balanced it relieves pressure on the back and even relieves sciatic pain.	When this meridian is balanced we feel more serene, relaxed and patient. We feel the opposite when the meridian is unbalanced (impatient, unable to relax, feeling pressure, intolerant, angry).
Liver	Used to transport Qi and blood through the body. The Liver meridian regulates blood pressure, helps keep a healthy back, and relieves abdominal pain.	Responsible for control and planning of bodily functions, the Liver meridian helps with feeling happy and trustful – which means it can be related to anger and aggression when not in balance.

Meridian	Physical benefit	Mental/emotional benefit
Gallbladder	The main function of this meridian is to control the flow of bile and help digestion by breaking down fats. It also helps get rid of toxins. No Gallbladder? No problem. TCM traces the meridian lines, even if the organ has been removed.	Known as the meridian of kindness, judgement, and decision making. When out of balance, it can lead of overstimulation, bitterness, and dislike.
Spleen	Helping with digestion, the Spleen helps sift food and blood moving them upward to the heart. It warms and transforms these into Qi (energy).	This meridian promotes thought and concentration. When the Spleen is out of balance, it can lead to worry, physical and mental stress, overeating (through stress), and chronic fatigue.
Stomach	Like the Spleen meridian, the Stomach meridian is a digestive organ responsible for absorbing nutrients and moving them downward. Reversing any partial blockage can relieve abdominal pain, a bloated feeling, and reflux disorder.	This comes as no surprise but when the Stomach meridian is balanced, we feel content, happy, and fulfilled. The opposite is true if the meridian doesn't function optimally. We feel hunger, greed, discontent, and disappointment.

MERIDIAN LINES

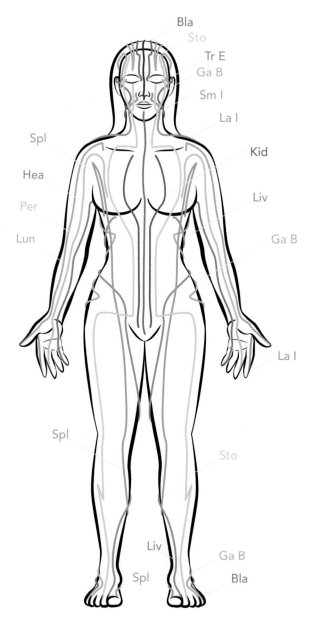

Bla
Sto
Tr E
Ga B
Sm I
La I

Spl
Kid
Hea
Per
Liv
Lun

Ga B

La I

Spl
Sto

Liv
Ga B
Spl
Bla

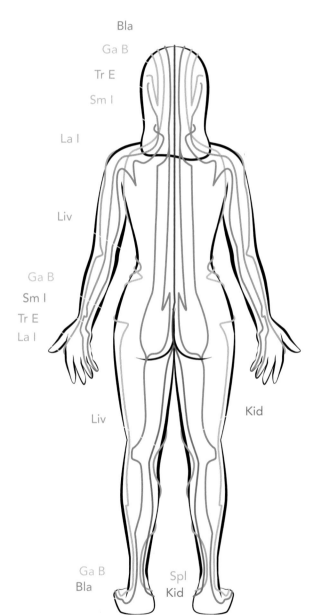

Bla
Ga B
Tr E
Sm I

La I

Liv

Ga B
Sm I
Tr E
La I

Liv

Kid

Ga B
Bla

Spl
Kid

TWO CENTERLINE MERIDIANS

• Conception Vessel
• **Governing Vessel**

TWELVE PRINCIPAL MERIDIANS

• Stomach Meridian
• Spleen Meridian

• Small Intestine Meridian
• Heart Meridian

• Bladder Meridian
• **Kidney Meridian**

• Pericadium Meridian
• Triple Energizer Meridian

• Gall Bladder Meridian
• Liver Meridian

• Lung Meridian
• Large Intestine Meridian

Other meridians, the upper body meridians:

The Heart meridian is said to control the flow of blood through the other organs – just as in Western medicine. When it is strong, it controls your emotions. When it is weak, your emotions control you.

The Small Intestine meridian receives food from the stomach that is partially digested and refines it even further. This meridian influences our immune system, growth, metabolism, and sexuality. When it is out of balance, it affects your judgment and clarity.

The Large Intestine meridian receives digested food and gets rid of it through body waste. It removes toxins and by-products from our bodies. If you like, it judges what stays and what goes. It governs emotions in the same way, helping us know when to let go. In TCM, emotions aren't about being good or bad, they are a feedback mechanism that shows your state of balance or disharmony in your body.

The Lung meridian assists with the circulation of breath, blood, and energy. As they say, "where blood goes, energy flows," which is true for breathing exercises when we practice yin yoga. The lung also regulates temperature and protects us from colds and flu. It helps with our self-esteem, and can make us sad, shameful, anxious, and sorrowful if it gets blocked.

The Pericardium meridian is not recognized in Western medicine, but its function is to protect the heart from damage. It helps regulate circulation through the blood vessels running from the heart. Pericardium energy helps with loving feelings associated with sex. It combines the raw sexual energy from the kidneys with love generated by the heart. In other words, it regulates joy and pleasure (or lack of if it's blocked).

The Triple Energizer meridian is another meridian that doesn't exist in Western medicine. It controls our fight-flight-or-freeze response. It's the only meridian not associated to a physical organ yet covers three parts: the chest for respiration and distributing energy, the diaphragm for digestion and pushing energy further, and to the top of the pubic bone for eliminating waste. It's said that when Triple Energizers are full, people can become more relaxed and kind-hearted. But activating the Triple Energizer can put us on high alert, releasing cortisol, and stressing our minds and bodies. It can even lead us to take on too much, or even eat more than we need to.

TCM. BELIEVE IT. OR NOT?

Meridian theory has its roots from China, India, Japan, and Tibet. Lately, Western medicine has dominated our thinking. But Western medicine looks purely at a symptom and treats that symptom. Headache? Take a pill. Feet swelling? Try some ointment. Hip pain? Here's a new hip. One thing about these traditional views of medicine is that they all see the importance of a holistic view of our minds and bodies.

So what can we believe? And what's best? While many scientists say that there is no evidence to support meridian theory, researchers at Seoul National University in Korea think they have found the existence of meridians. They call them the "primo-vascular system," a part of the cardiovascular system. They discovered that meridian lines are not confined to the skin, but are a duct system where liquid flows, and that this liquid forms stem cells.

ACUPRESSURE AND ACUPUNCTURE

Each meridian has acupressure (or acupuncture – inserting a needle) points running along its line. Studies have shown that acupuncture is effective for a variety of conditions. According to the World Health Organization, acupuncture is used in 103 of 129 countries that reported data.

How acupuncture works is not fully understood. But there's evidence that acupuncture may have effects on the nervous system and on other body tissues.

Acupuncture seems to be particularly effective in treating pain. The NCCIH analysis of data from 20 studies referenced in the previous chapter (6,376 participants) of people with painful conditions (back pain, osteoarthritis, neck pain, or headaches) showed that the beneficial effects of acupuncture continued for a year after the end of treatment for all conditions except neck pain.

When we practice yin yoga, we stimulate these points through gently putting pressure on those meridian lines – acupressure. In other words, we can go some way to reproducing the effects of acupuncture when we practice yin yoga.

Let's get STARTED

You know why you should be doing yin yoga, so let's look at the how. There are two phrases about yoga in general and yin yoga specifically that you should take to heart.

It's your body. It's your yoga

No two people are the same – especially as we age. So what one person can do, maybe another can't. What matters is that you regularly use the poses in this section to stretch and release your connective tissues, loosening up tight muscles and sore joints.

You don't use your body to get into the pose. You use the pose to get into your body

Who cares if you don't look like that stretchy, bendy person who can fold in more ways than an origami figure? What matters is being in a state of physical and mental awareness where you feel that you're doing yourself good. You are stretching your body and you're feeling the benefit.

At the same time, you're concentrating on giving yourself that "me time," that mental and emotional stillness where you can leave our fast-paced information overloaded world behind for just a few minutes. The physical, mental, and emotional effects are very rewarding.

Find your edge

As we talked about with the Goldilocks philosophy, finding your edge is finding the level of a pose that's right for just you. While you should feel tension from the pose you are in, you should feel you can hold the pose for a longer time – around three minutes or longer as you practice more.

You'll find your edge widens over time, so if you can't stretch your leg fully on the floor when doing a pose, you probably will by the end of the time you are in the pose.

Find stillness

If we can stay still in a pose, we allow our bodies to get the full benefit of what we are doing. Being still doesn't mean playing statues, it means trying to relax into the pose and letting gravity do its work. During the time you hold the pose you'll feel your body unlocking as you add a few extra millimeters to your stretch.

But it's not just our bodies that benefit. Finding stillness gives us the opportunity to listen to our minds. Use the time and the stillness to give yourself space. Relax and rewind – even with your tissues under tension. Use your breathing to get comfortable and contemplative. Check out the advice on breathing later in the book.

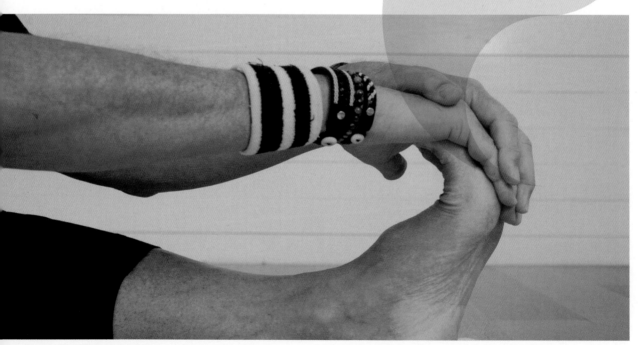

Find time

The recommended time to hold a yin yoga pose is from three minutes upward. Whenever you need physiotherapy the therapist will often tell you to stay in a stretch for some time. The benefit is obvious, the longer you hold, the deeper the stretch. The more you stretch, the more your connective tissues can "give." The more they give, the better you feel, as your body pulls itself back into shape.

Think about the hours you sit in front of a screen, or on the sofa bingeing another few episodes or games. Slouching with your neck forward. This is your chance to correct the damage.

If three minutes seems like too long in the beginning, fine. Come out of the pose and relax. Any stretch for more than a minute has benefits.

Remember: If you feel pain, stop if it hurts, adjust the pose, or come out altogether and just lie comfortably until you feel it's time to try another pose.

Breathing is natural. Right? But it's often regulated unconsciously. If we are stressed then we breathe too fast and too heavily for our own good. And stress is probably the number one killer in the Western world.

We all know the medical conditions related to stress, from heart attacks and strokes to mental imbalances, reduced immune system, diabetes, and cancer. One way of helping relieve stress is through better breathing techniques.

Breathing in a controlled way helps balance energy, puts you in a better mood, and increases your concentration.

Here are three types of breathing that help you with your yoga practice, and help you relieve stress.

Ocean breathing (Ujjayi breathing)

The simplest way to explain ocean breathing is to imagine you are cleaning your sunglasses. You'd breathe out and probably make a sound. Another way to describe it is to breathe out and make what you think is the sound of the ocean. The idea of ocean breathing (like other types of yoga breathing or pranayama breathing) is to breathe a lot of air into and out of your lungs to calm your system.

Abdominal breathing

Put your right hand over your heart and your left hand over your navel and take in deep breaths through your nose and expel the air through your mouth. The trick is to expand your stomach so it's larger than your chest (unless your stomach is already larger than your chest).

Alternative nostril breathing

Slowly breathe in and out, then close your right nostril with your right thumb. Take a big breath in through your left nostril. Now release your thumb and block your left nostril. Breathe out from your right nostril. Try this a few times on each side.

4x4 breathing

This breathing exercise is probably the best 4x4 by far. Count to four as you breathe in, then count to four as you expel air through your mouth. A nice way to relax is to exhale for longer than your count of four.

The sympathetic and parasympathetic nervous systems are the parts of our nervous system that regulate our involuntary body functions. The sympathetic system controls our fight-or-flight responses. It kicks in as soon as we feel threatened. It is also the system that builds cortisol that can lead to stress.

The parasympathetic system controls our rest-and-digest system. It slows down some responses, making the body feel calm, allowing it to rest, relax, and repair itself. Yin yoga activates our parasympathetic systems, calming our bodies and minds.

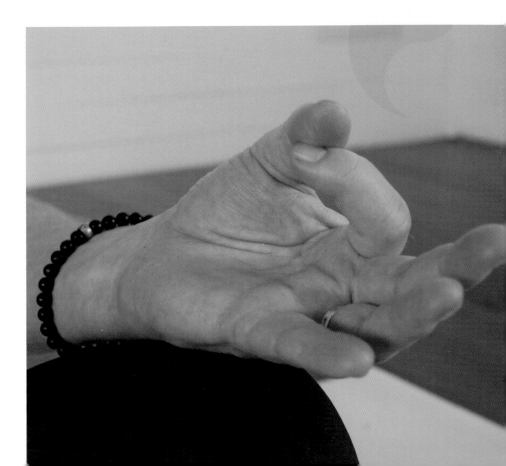

PROPS FOR GREATER COMFORT AND SUPPORT

Where are you stiff most? And what areas of your body do you want to unlock? Using the right props lets you stay in certain poses much more comfortably and holding them for longer, meaning you can get more benefit and a stronger, more flexible, healthier body – and mind.

Here's a list of the main props you can use for yin yoga. But the bottom line is, if you have a blanket, or two, you can practice where you want to, when you want to.

Mat. A proper yoga mat makes you more comfortable and acts as a barrier between you and the floor. I'd recommend buying a thicker mat to give you more support for sensitive areas like your knees, elbows, or your feet.

Blocks. These help you by supporting you in different positions, like propping your hands and arms, sitting on them, raising your body, and can even be used between your legs to keep them together. I find blocks are a great way to make the poses suit my body so I can stay in the pose for longer.

Blankets. A nice thick blanket adds more support and comfort to your practice. Rest your head, support your feet – and add extra comfort to all areas in between. Use a blanket to keep warm and snug when you are relaxing before and after your session.

Bolster. These big, comfortable pillows are perfect for supporting joints when you sit or lie on them. They provide more comfort so you can hold poses for longer.

Straps. Use straps to pull your feet closer to your body, or pull yourself down to bring your head closer to your knees. You could put together a complete routine using straps.

Remember that the purpose of yin yoga is to help you relax. So while you can wear any type of clothing for your practice, you'll be more comfortable in loose-fitting clothing, and maybe an extra layer or blanket to keep you nice and warm.

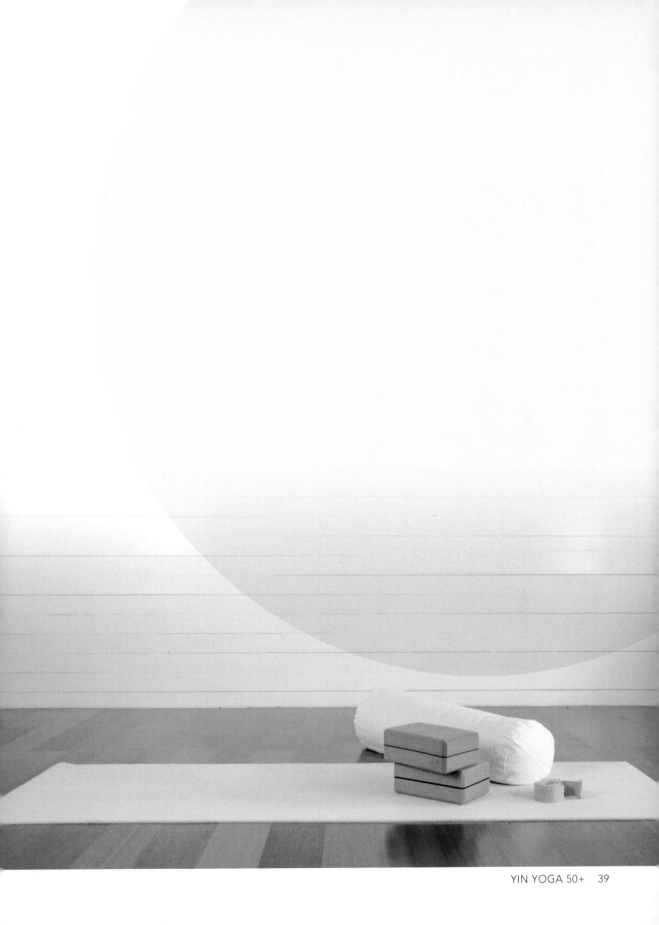

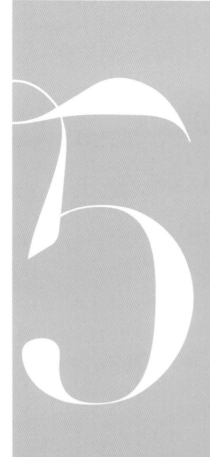

Strike a pose

YIN YOGA ASANAS THAT ARE PERFECT FOR PEOPLE AGED 50+

Some yin yoga poses (asanas) are easier than others, but all of them offer benefits to your health and wellbeing. This section shows you the major yin yoga poses with suggestions about the best way of doing them, how to make them easier if you need to, and what counterposes to do after each pose.

WHEN AND HOW TO PRACTICE

Any time is a good time to get on the floor and stretch. But two excellent times are early in the morning when our muscles are still a bit sleepy (and probably stiff), and before you go to bed, allowing you to relax more and calm your nervous system for a longer, deeper, more restful sleep.

I recommend closing your eyes during poses, as it allows you to get rid of some of the "noise" of what's going on around you and think inward to your body. But it's entirely up to you if you want your eyes open or not.

BRING BACK YOUR AWARENESS

You're holding yin yoga poses for a relatively long time. So if (when) your mind starts to wander, try to concentrate on your body, on the sensations you're feeling. If you feel stiffness in a particular area—say your left hip—concentrate on directing your breathing to that point. That way you can send energy to it, helping release your whole body.

If you're struggling with concentration, don't worry. Let your thoughts slide into your mind, then slide out. Try to concentrate on your breathing.

Remember, where concentration goes, energy flows.

EVERY POSE HAS ITS COUNTERPOSE

Enjoy a rest, say up to one minute, after every pose to let your body react to the stressing and stretching you've just subjected it to. Then it's a good idea to add a counterpose–stretching your body in the opposite direction. Counterposes return your body to its natural condition so you don't carry the tensions from one stretch into another.

The result? Stronger, more supple bodies.

MUSIC—THE FOOD OF LOVE— AND THE PERFECT YOGA SEDATIVE

Doing yin yoga poses on your own is a great way to a healthy life of better physicality and lower levels of stress. Adding the right music, that is low-level, slow, and relaxing will add to your practice, letting you release, relax, and let go. You'll find lots of playlists on all common music streaming sites.

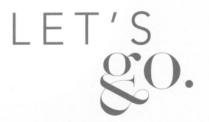

LET'S go.

Ankle stretch

WHY IT'S GOOD FOR YOU

This is a tough pose that stretches the muscles, ligaments, and tendons in your ankles, keeping your leg strong and flexible. It improves your flexibility and range of motion which helps with your balance. It increases blood circulation to the entire foot including your toes, protects the ankle joint, and avoids injury.

Still running or walking a lot? Ankle Stretch helps keep the muscles in good condition, preventing injury, allowing you to run (or walk) for years to come.

HOW TO DO IT

Sit on your heels, lean back, and try to lift your knees off the floor. Allow your knees to lift as much as is comfortable for you.

Note: This pose can put a lot of strain on your ankles and knees. If it hurts, come out and sit in Child's pose, which also gives your ankles a gentle stretch.

Spend about one minute in the pose. Longer if you can.

TIP

Millimeters matter. This pose can be uncomfortable, so try for around a minute at first. As with all poses, each time you stretch, you add those important millimeters to your total range of motion.

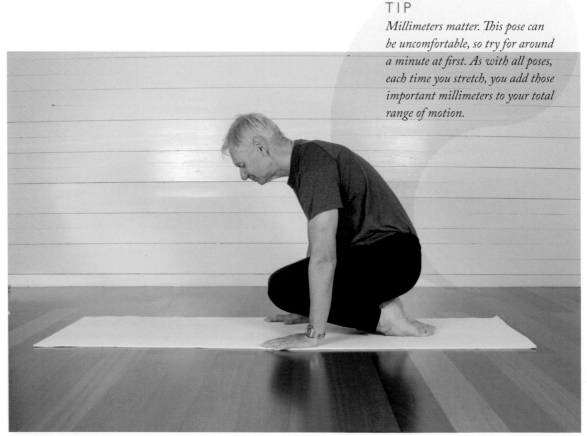

THE EASIER WAY

Put a blanket in the crease of your knees, which will make the pose more comfortable. You can even rest your knees on a bolster.

COUNTERPOSE

Press-up pose or Plank pose, both of which flex your feet in the opposite direction.

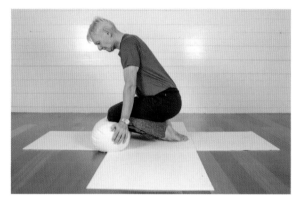

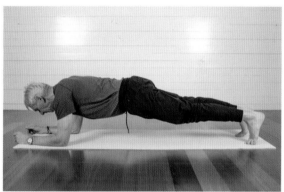

COMING OUT OF THE POSE

Lean forward and bring your hands in front of your knees. Maybe stay in a Tabletop position for a while to relax.

The physio says... This pose stimulates your big toe and increases balance, which helps in having the right gait when you're walking. This can offset mobility issues.

Meridians

This pose stimulates all lower meridians as they all flow through the feet.

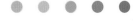

Bananasana

WHY IT'S GOOD FOR YOU

Super for people 50+, Bananasana stretches your shoulders, arms, chest, core, and lower back.

It stresses the IT (iliotibial) band, relieving pressure on your knee joints. Tight IT bands often result in "runner's knee" and lots of associated knee problems.

Bananasana helps with breathing by stretching the intercostal muscles around your ribcage.

HOW TO DO IT

Lie down in Savasana (Corpse pose) with your hands by your sides. To stretch your left side, bring your bottom to the left-hand side of your mat.

Bring your hands over your head and stretch out fully.

Keep your feet together and move them to the right. If you prefer, cross your left foot over your right foot.

Grab your left wrist with your right hand then gently pull.

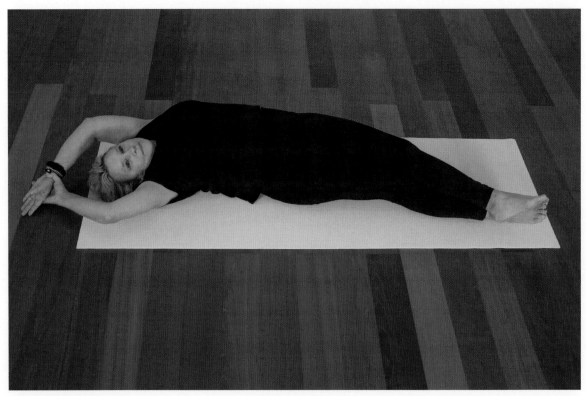

Try to stay relaxed and don't put too much pressure on your lower back.

Be careful with your arms when you come out of the pose. Bring them slowly back to your sides.

To stretch your right side, bring your bottom to the right side of the mat and repeat the instructions in reverse.

The physio says... Lots of pain at the side of your back is a result of you being tight on one or both sides. This pose helps rectify this and alleviate back pain.

TIP

As the saying goes, if you're feeling it, you're doing it. You know you're making a difference to your body. Maybe adjust your edge after you've been in a pose for a while?

THE EASIER WAY

If you have a problem with your shoulders you can simply keep your arms by your sides. Alternatively, you don't have to cross your feet over.

COMING OUT OF THE POSE

Just bring your arms back down by your sides, uncouple your feet if you've crossed them and relax in Savasana.

COUNTERPOSE

An excellent counterpose is to hug your knees to your chest. Keep your head and shoulders on the mat to avoid stressing them.

Either rock from side to side to give your back a massage, or alternatively stretch out one leg and then the other, pulling your other leg close to your body.

Meridians

Stimulates the Liver and Gallbladder meridians, helping digestion.

Bridge

WHY IT'S GOOD FOR YOU

Bridge pose tones both your spine and back. It helps relieve pain in your hips, while stretching your arms and shoulders. It helps tone your stomach muscles too.

Regulating the flow of blood to the heart, Bridge pose is good for your blood pressure and helps improve digestion.

HOW TO DO IT

Come into Bridge pose by placing your feet flat on the floor with your knees bent.

Place your arms down by your side with palms facing down and walk your heels up until they meet your fingers. Lift your hips up and slide a block under your bottom. Make sure your block is under your pelvis and not your lower back.

Now slide your legs down so that you feel the tension from the block. If you want, you can stretch your arms over your head for a deeper stretch.

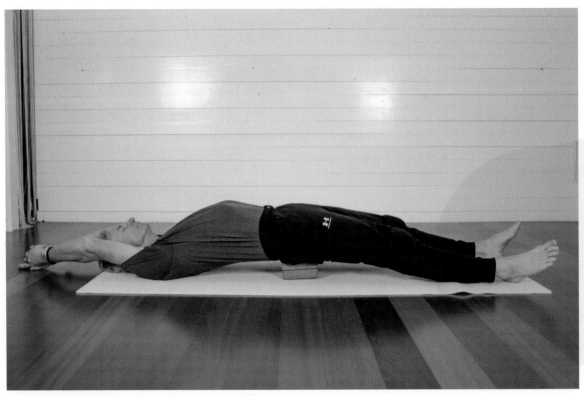

NEED MORE?

Once you've found your edge, you may want to increase the stress. Simply slide another block under the first one. Make sure to use the flat side of the blocks so they don't fall while you are in the pose.

COUNTERPOSE

Hug your knees to your chest, keeping your head and shoulders on the floor. Maybe roll from side to side to massage your back?

TIP
Keep your eyes closed and use slow, deep breathing to relax deeper into this, or any yin yoga pose.

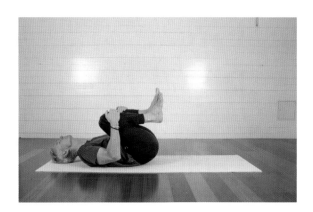

COMING OUT OF THE POSE

If you've raised your arms, bring them back down by your sides. Bring up your knees and push on your feet to raise your bottom of the block, then slide it away while you slide down to the floor. Relax.

The physio says... This pose stretches the chest muscles and relieves tension in your shoulders and back. It also helps us to breathe better.

Meridians

Bridge pose stimulates several meridians including Kidney and Bladder, Spleen and Stomach, and the Heart meridians.

Butterfly/RECLINING BUTTERFLY

WHY IT'S GOOD FOR YOU

Butterfly stretches your hips, knee joints, pelvis, shoulders, and neck. It stretches your lower back, even if your hamstrings are tight.

The physio says... Hips become tight, especially in men. This pose relieves pressure on your glutes and hips.

TIP
If your groin complains, just stretch out your arms and legs to make yourself as long as possible.

HOW TO DO IT

Bring the soles of your feet together and let your knees fall either side toward the floor. Don't try to force your knees, just find your edge. Allow your back to fold forward and try to relax.

Bulging discs? Keep straight as you come forward rather than round your back.

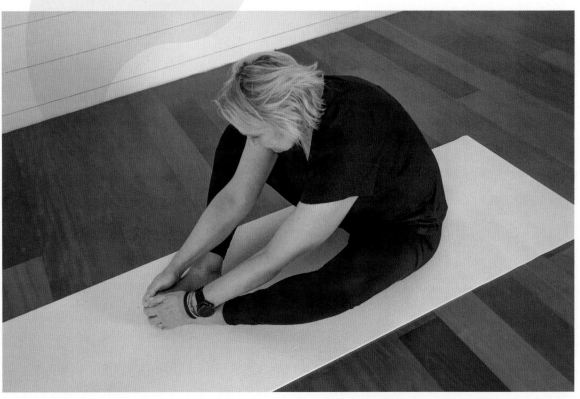

RECLINING BUTTERFLY

From a lying position, bring your knees up and have them flat on the floor. Now put the soles of your feet together and let your knees fall either side toward the floor. Don't try to force your knees, just find your edge.

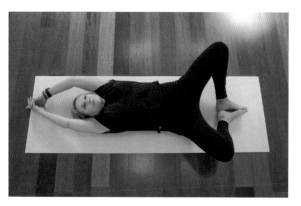

Try lifting your arms above your head and resting them on the floor to stretch your shoulders and your upper and lower back.

THE EASIER WAY

Use a block, sit cushion, or blanket to sit on. If your bones feel supported, your muscles relax.

COMING OUT OF THE POSE

Straighten up your back until you're upright. If you need to, push your knees gently with your hands until they come together. Now lie down and relax. If you're in Reclining Butterfly, bring your arms down by your sides first.

COUNTERPOSE

Teepee. Put your feet flat on the floor on the edge of your mat with your knees pointing upward. Now push your knees together.

Window Wipers. From the Teepee position, start to roll your legs down to one side of your mat as far as

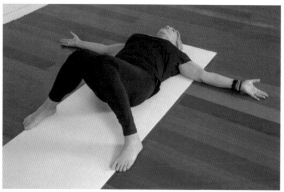

you can, then up again. Now sink them to the other side. Do as many turns as you like.

Meridians

Butterfly pose affects the Gallbladder, Kidney, Liver, and Bladder meridians.

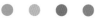

Cat Pulling its Tail

WHY IT'S GOOD FOR YOU

This is an excellent pose to stimulate your feet, ankle, knee, quadriceps, lower back, spine, and oblique muscles in your stomach.

The physio says... This pose will relieve pressure on your back by stretching the hip flexors and surrounding muscles.

HOW TO DO IT

Lie on your right side with your body along the side of your mat. Bend your knees to ninety degrees.

Support your head with your palm or against the side of your arm.

Bring your left leg forward and to the side over your right leg. Now grab your bottom (right) foot and pull it toward your buttocks.

Reverse the sequence for the other side.

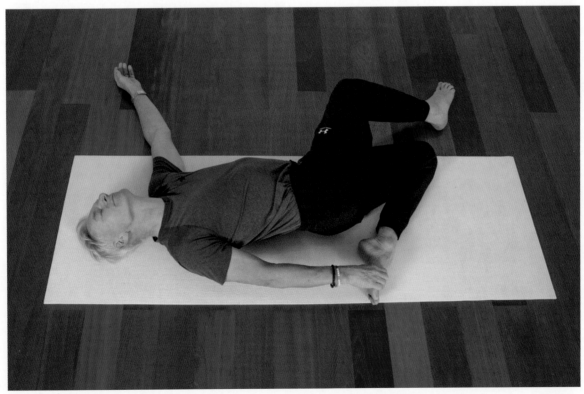

THE EASIER WAY

If you feel too much tightness by pulling your bottom leg, leave it and enjoy the side bend.

COMING OUT OF THE POSE

Just let go of your ankle and bring your left leg back, relaxing back into a lying position.

COUNTERPOSE

Child's pose (see description) or hug your knees to your chest.

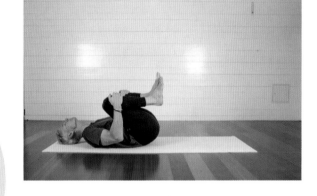

TIP

Accept your body for what it is. Try to release your muscles by letting go of any distractions. Keep your eyes closed and think inward.

Meridians

Stimulates the Stomach and Spleen, Bladder, and Kidney meridians.

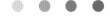

Caterpillar/DANGLING

WHY IT'S GOOD FOR YOU

Caterpillar (and Dangling) stretches and compresses the tendons and tissues around your spine and abdomen. It's an excellent stretch for your hamstrings.

The physio says... This exercises stretches the hamstrings, taking pressure off our lower backs, often alleviating pain.

HOW TO DO IT

Caterpillar
Sit on a block or cushion. Push both legs out in front of you and try to straighten them as much as you can. Now fold forward, bending your back. Maybe trace your fingers down your quads, knees, and tops of your calves to find your edge?

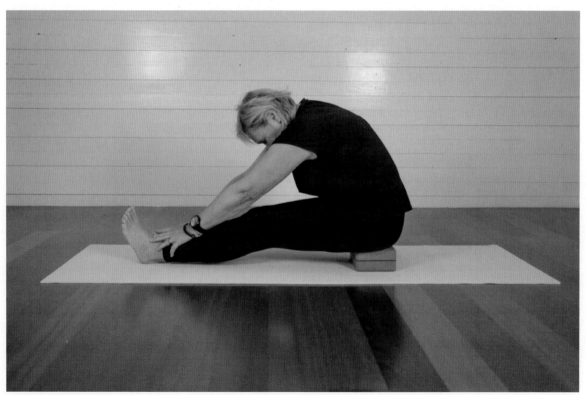

HOW TO DO IT

Dangling
From standing, fold forward, pushing your hands down the front of your legs until you feel your edge.

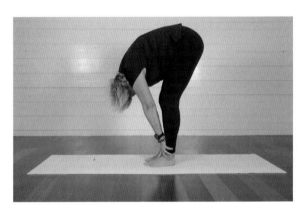

THE EASIER WAY

You might have problems straightening your legs. Sit on a cushion or block and straighten your legs as much as you can. Sitting up straight rather than bending forward might be easier.

COMING OUT OF THE POSE

Use your hands to slowly push yourself up to a sitting position. Push up from a standing position if you've been in Dangling pose.

COUNTERPOSE

Lean back onto your elbows, keep your feet together and move them from side to side to release any tension in your spine or stomach.

TIP

Let gravity do the work. You'll find your knees come closer to the floor over time while you're in the pose. And of course, the more you do it, the more flexible you become.

Meridians

Stimulates the
Bladder meridian.

●

Child's pose

WHY IT'S GOOD FOR YOU

This pose is a classic counterpose for many other poses, but a great pose to do every day. It gently stretches out your spine, thighs, hips, and ankles and helps relieve back and neck pain. It's also a great pose to soothe and calm as it stimulates the flow of blood to your head.

The physio says... When your back muscles are tight, they can easily tire and weaken, leading to problems. Child's pose is a great way to relax the whole body's structure, potentially preventing that damage.

HOW TO DO IT

From a Tabletop position, put your toes together and keep your knees a hip-width apart. Now push back until your bottom comes back between your knees – or as far back as you can go to find your edge.

Extend your arms in front of you with your head on the mat or on a blanket (on the mat).

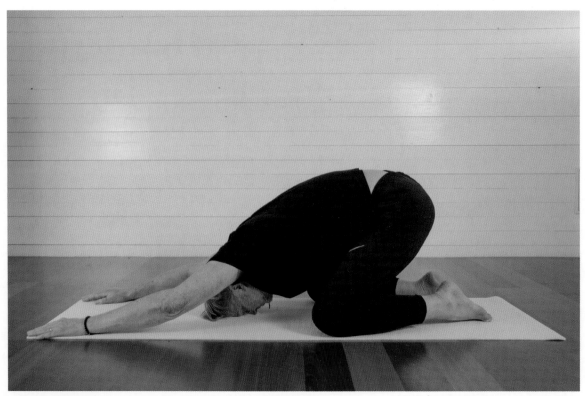

THE EASIER WAY

Maybe have your legs wider apart? And if it's more comfortable, have your arms along the sides of your body.

COUNTERPOSE

Child's pose is often used as a counterpose. But if you've been in the pose for several minutes, then rocking backward and forward in Tabletop position is a great loosener.

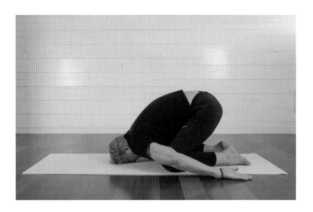

TIP

Don't try to use your body to get into the pose—use the pose to get into your body. Don't care what other people look like, just focus on the benefit you're giving yourself.

COMING OUT OF THE POSE

Push up with your bottom and arms until you come back into Tabletop position.

Meridians

Stimulates Kidney, Bladder, and Spleen meridians. Keeping your knees wide apart targets the Liver meridian.

Deer

WHY IT'S GOOD FOR YOU

Deer pose is a gentle pose that helps with external and internal rotation of your hips. It also gives you a gentle upper body twist. It engages the lower back muscles, glutes, knees, quads, and even your neck. It's thought to be a great pose to help lower back issues like sciatica and piriformis syndrome.

The physio says... There is a theory that hip rotation in poses like Deer pose stimulate the fascia, aiding flexibility.

HOW TO DO IT

Either start in Butterfly or have your legs straight out in front of you.

Let your right knee come up then try to lay it flat on the floor in front of you.

Now bend your left knee and pull it slightly so that both knees mirror each other. Try to keep your sitting bones on the floor.

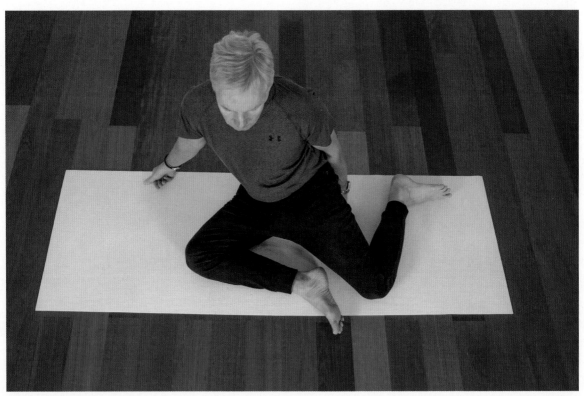

THE EASIER WAY

Maybe lean forward or sideways onto a bolster for a relaxing back stretch.

COUNTERPOSE

One side is a counterpose to the other, but Window Wipers is an excellent way to loosen the hips and legs after stretching each side.

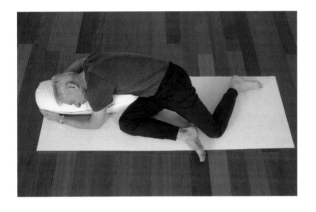

TIP

Remember, you shouldn't feel pain. Once you're in the pose, try to direct your breath to where you feel most tension so that you can stay in the pose for longer, maximizing the benefit.

COMING OUT OF THE POSE

Lean toward your forward leg then swing your back foot forward until your knees are together. Roll around to a sitting position.

Meridians

Stimulates the Gallbladder, Kidney, and Liver meridians.

Dragon

WHY IT'S GOOD FOR YOU

Dragon poses open your hip and groin and stretch your glutes. They also target the hip flexors and quads in your rear leg. Dragon poses may even help with sciatic pain by relieving tightness in your legs and hips.

The physio says... This pose releases the hip flexors. It helps the lower back relax, helping prevent damage.

HOW TO DO IT

There are several different types of Dragon pose. Here I suggest you try Inside Dragon.

Go into a Tabletop position. Step your right leg forward until you feel your back (left leg) is flexed. Now put your hands inside your right leg.

TIP
Yin yoga stimulates your rest and digest system (parasympathetic system). It reduces cortisol, and consequently stress, regulates your heartbeat and helps you relax.

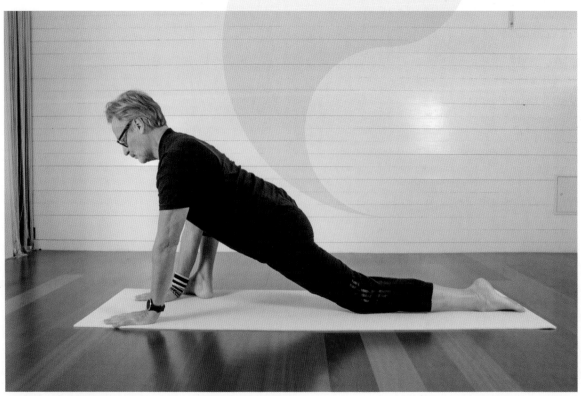

WANT MORE?

Go down onto your elbows or push against the side of your right leg. Maybe straighten your rear leg by lifting your knee off the floor for the last minute of the pose? This is called Fire-Breathing Dragon.

THE EASIER WAY

From Tabletop, step your right leg out until your left leg is flexed. Now simply rest your arms on your front (right) knee for support. This is Dragon Flying High.

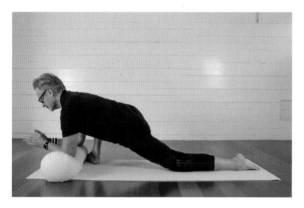

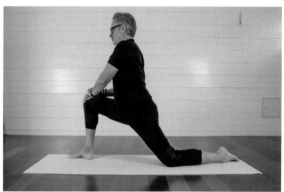

COMING OUT OF THE POSE

Just step your front foot back and slowly come back to Tabletop.

COUNTERPOSE

Gently rock backward and forward on your hands and knees to release any tension in your body.

Meridians

Dragon poses target the Stomach, Spleen, Liver, Gallbladder, Kidney, and Bladder meridians.

Frog

WHY IT'S GOOD FOR YOU

An excellent hip opener, Frog pose also stretches your groin, inner thighs, and core muscles. As you're in a forward bend it can even stretch your chest and shoulders. It also activates the pelvis, glutes, and hamstrings, increasing your flexibility and range of motion.

The physio says... Your adductor (groin) muscles become stiff and can create groin and hip problems. This pose helps release tension, especially around the groin.

HOW TO DO IT

Begin in Tabletop position on your hands and knees. Now open your hips and turn your feet outward to the sides.

Lower yourself onto your forearms. Push your hips backward until you feel a deep stretch in your hips and inner thighs. Only go as far as your edge.

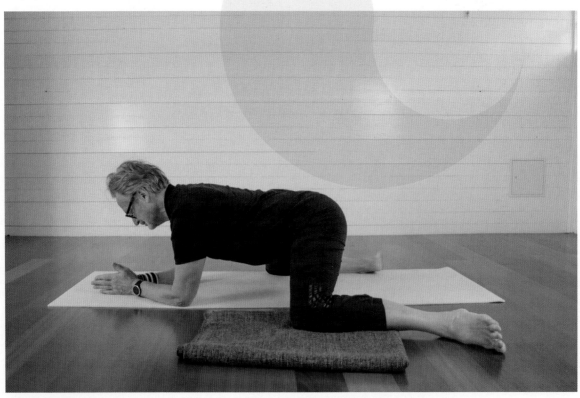

THE EASIER WAY

Keep your knees closer together, like in Child's pose, or do the supported half Frog pose. Lie on a bolster with your legs straight, then bring up one leg at a time. This is a nice restorative stretch.

COUNTERPOSE

Either go into Child's pose or lie on your back and hug your knees to your chest.

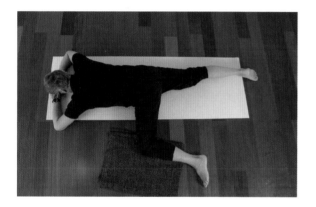

TIP
Scan your body both before and after each practice. Which parts were sore and aching before you started? How do they feel after you've finished?

COMING OUT OF THE POSE

Slowly push your knees closer together until you come into Tabletop.

Meridians

Spleen, Liver and Kidney. If you stretch your arms out you activate the Heart and Lung meridians.

Half Butterfly

WHY IT'S GOOD FOR YOU

If you don't do any other pose, do this one regularly.
You can do one side at a time while you watch the
TV adverts. Half Butterfly stretches the hamstrings
of your extended leg and the inner thigh, groin, and
knee of your folded leg. The folded leg also stretches
your hip flexors, which can relieve pain and tension
on the hips and knees. Folding forward stretches your
spine.

HOW TO DO IT

Sit on a block or cushion, bend one leg and draw your
foot into your inner leg. If you want to stretch your
adductors (groin), bring your foot closer to the top of
your leg. If you want to stretch your hamstrings, bring
your foot closer to your knee.

Now fold forward over your straight leg to the front,
or to the side. Turn your torso toward the center.

TIP

*If you have a watch that measures your pulse, check your
pulse level when you start and after you finish your yin
yoga session. You'll be surprised at the difference.*

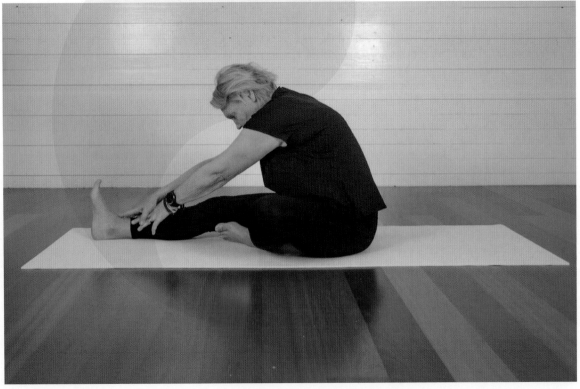

THE EASIER WAY

Place a cushion under your knee if you have problems with your knees or if you have tight hamstrings, or lie down and do the pose on the wall.

COUNTERPOSE

Window Wipers or lie on your back and cradle your knees.

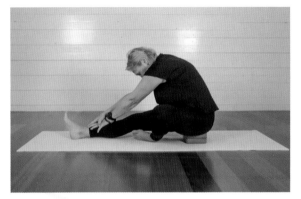

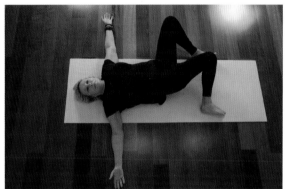

COMING OUT OF THE POSE

Straighten your bent leg then slowly push your body up to sitting.

Meridians

Stretching your hips and inside leg stimulates the Kidney, Liver, Gallbladder, and Bladder meridians.

Happy Baby

WHY IT'S GOOD FOR YOU

Happy Baby stretches your hamstrings, hips, groin, abdomen, calves, triceps, and chest. It can realign your spine, helping relieve back pain by stretching the surrounding muscles, tendons, and ligaments.

The physio says... This is an excellent pose to stimulate your glutes—your biggest muscles—and help relax your back.

HOW TO DO IT

Lie on your back and grab your knees, hugging them to your chest. If you can, get hold of the soles of your feet.

Keeping your head and shoulders on the floor, pull your knees to the floor.

TIP
Try to keep your eyes closed during the poses to concentrate on the parts of your body you are trying to affect. It really is a case of mind over matter. And you're what matters!

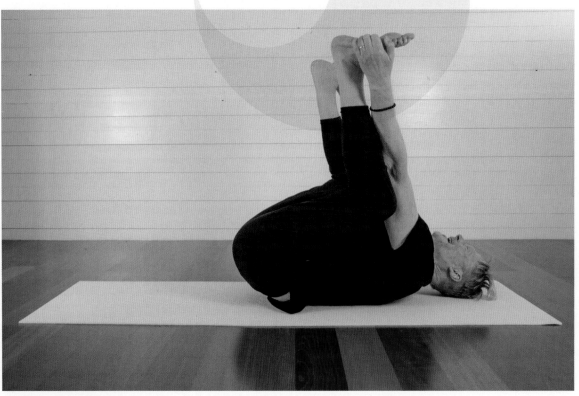

THE EASIER WAY

Hold onto your ankles, shins, or knees, or even use a belt under the soles of your feet.

COUNTERPOSE

Window Wipers or move your legs from side to side.

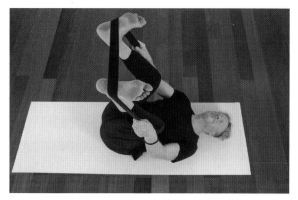

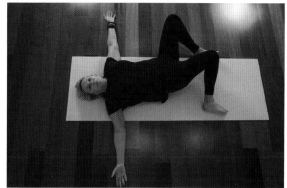

COMING OUT OF THE POSE

Let go of your feet/shins/knees and let your legs slowly fall onto the ground into Savasana.

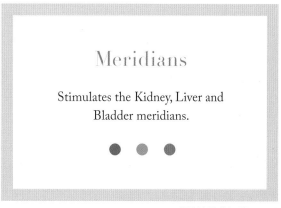

Meridians

Stimulates the Kidney, Liver and Bladder meridians.

● ● ●

Melting Heart

WHY IT'S GOOD FOR YOU

Melting Heart is a great way to open up and relax your upper back (latissimus dorsi), shoulders, and neck. It stretches the middle part of your spine, helping you get a better posture. You also stimulate your stomach muscles.

The physio says... This pose adds the double effect of opening up your chest and stretching the latissimus muscles of your upper back. It's a great antidote for desk jockeys.

HOW TO DO IT

Start off in Tabletop position (on all fours). Keep your knees a little wider than hip-distance apart, then come down onto your elbows.

Keeping your hips in line with your knees, push your arms in front of you, one after the other, until they are stretched out as far as possible.

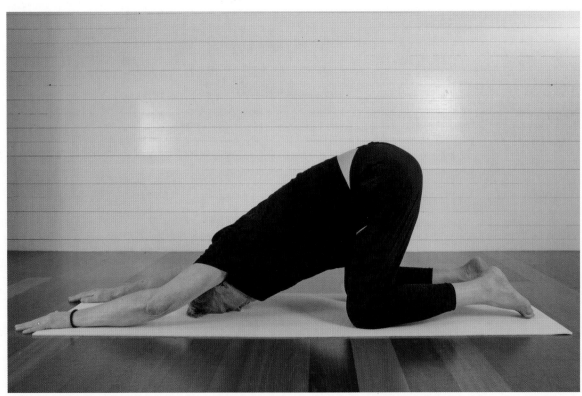

THE EASIER WAY

If you feel a tingling sensation or you have a problem stretching your shoulders right out, back out of the pose a little or stretch out one arm at a time.

COUNTERPOSE

Flapping Fish is an excellent counterpose that stresses the shoulder blade of your extended arm, releasing any tension. It can help to reduce lower back pain and aid digestion.

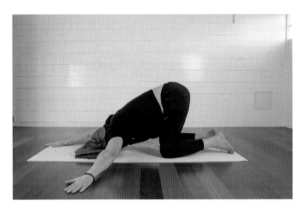

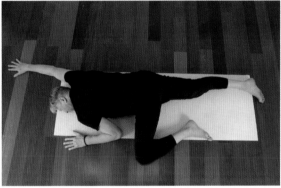

COMING OUT OF THE POSE

Slowly push backward until you come back into Tabletop.

To get into Flapping Fish, lower your bent shoulder onto the mat and keep your arm straight. Remember to breathe in a slow, harmonic way.

TIP

As we get older our bodies become less symmetrical. Spend more time in poses on areas where you feel stiffer, bringing symmetry back. For instance if your right shoulder feels stiffer than your left, then spend more time with your right shoulder in this position.

Meridians

Stimulates the Bladder, Stomach and Spleen, Heart, and Lung meridians.

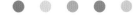

Open Wing

WHY IT'S GOOD FOR YOU

One of my favorite poses, Open Wing, opens your pectoral and bicep tissues and targets the deeper tissues of your shoulders. It releases tension, even in your hips and inner thighs. It puts gentle pressure on your upper arm which helps strengthen your biceps and triceps. I find this pose good for tennis elbow as I grip my golf clubs too hard.

The physio says... If the top of your chest muscles are tight, it can lead to problems with the shoulder. These are excellent poses to counteract the effects of this.

HOW TO DO IT

Lie on your stomach. Extend both your arms to 90 degrees.

To stretch your right side, look left, then lift your left arm close to the left shoulder. Bring up your left knee.

Use your left palm to lift your chest and regulate the stress on your right shoulder.

TIP
Think about being mindful: Live in the moment. Accept yourself. Focus on your breathing.

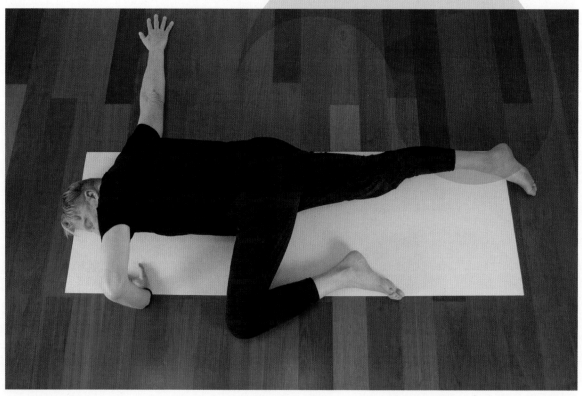

WANT MORE?

Bring your left leg over your body and plant it on your right side. More? Take your left arm over your back so it's parallel with your right arm.

COUNTERPOSE

Thread the Needle. Bring your right arm through your left arm from a Tabletop position.

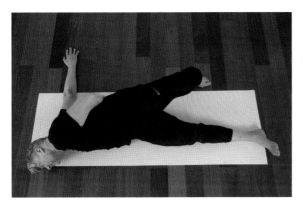

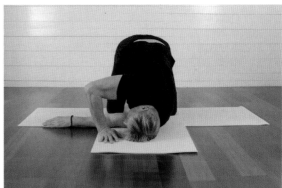

MAKE IT EASIER

Just don't push so hard with your palm. It's easy to regulate pressure, then increase it as your shoulder moves deeper over time.

COMING OUT OF THE POSE

Release your arm that's adding pressure, then slide your leg back so both legs are parallel and your arms are spread out.

Meridians

Stimulates the Stomach and Spleen meridians.

● ●

Saddle/Half Saddle

WHY IT'S GOOD FOR YOU

As I'm not too flexible, I find this a tough pose, but the effects are excellent. It's a great stretch for the sacrum, hip flexors, and quads as well as putting pressure on your ankles and lower legs. It helps bring back more mobility to your posture.

HOW TO DO IT

Lean backward with your heels spread wider than your knees, then lean back onto your hands. If you can go further, come down to your elbows. Even further? Put your back and your head on the floor.

TIP
If you find a pose is too uncomfortable, don't do it. There's always an alternative way to stretch and strengthen all areas of your body.

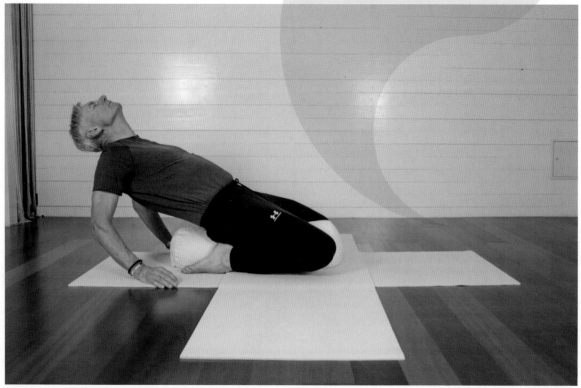

THE EASIER WAY

Do one leg at a time in a Half Saddle while sitting on a block or a bolster. Still too tough? Lie on your stomach, grab your heel or even your leg under your knee and pull as far as you can into your body.

COUNTERPOSE

Child's pose, or Plank/Push-up pose.

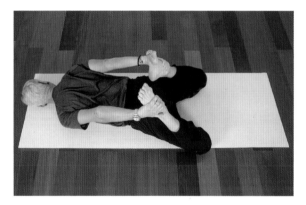

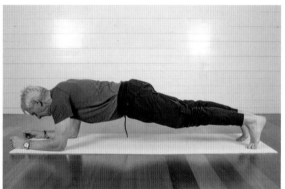

COMING OUT OF THE POSE

Push yourself up the way you came, or even turn to one side to release out of the pose.

Meridians

Stimulates the Stomach, Spleen, Bladder, and Kidney meridians.

Savasana (Corpse pose)

WHY IT'S GOOD FOR YOU

Time for a rest while calming your whole body? Savasana helps you move away from our stressful lives, to awakening the parasympathetic rest-and-digest response. It slows down our cardiovascular system, brings oxygen to the blood (with the right breathing), and gives us a greater awareness of our bodies. Quite simply it reduces anxiety—and your blood pressure— while promoting relaxation and healing.

HOW TO DO IT

Lie flat on your mat and maybe have a blanket or pillow under your head for support. Separate your legs and let them fall flat.

Keep your palms up to the ceiling or sky and just let your body relax into itself. Close your eyes and breathe slowly and deeply.

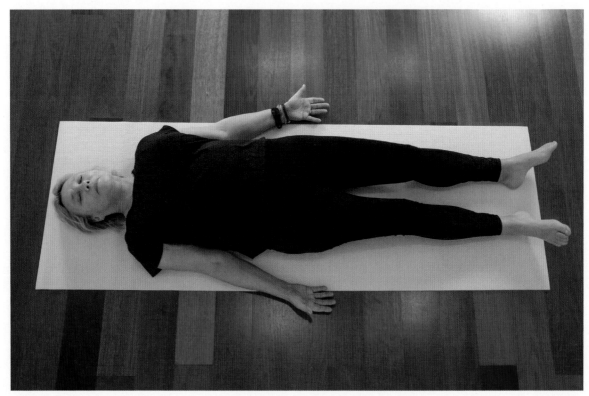

THE EASIER WAY

There isn't an easier way, although you might want to put a bolster under your knees for comfort, or even lie on a bolster to stretch out your shoulders.

COUNTERPOSE

Just do any pose you like after Savasana. I use it to start and finish every yin session.

TIP
Make Savasana a daily habit to calm and relax your body. And stay in the pose for around ten to twelve percent of the total time you practice yin yoga to really benefit.

Shoelace

WHY IT'S GOOD FOR YOU

Shoelace stretches the IT band and your glutes while targeting your hamstrings, inner thighs, and groins. Flexing the knee joint keeps the ligaments strong, helping prevent injury and arthritis.

The physio says... Some poses are more difficult than others for some people. Often this is simply because people's bone structure is different. Maybe you simply can't rotate as much as other people can.

HOW TO DO IT

I advise sitting on a blanket, block, or bolster.

From Butterfly pose, let your right knee fall onto the floor and maybe pull it closer to your left hip.

Cross your left leg over your right and stack your knees on top of each other if you can. Try to have both your sitting bones on the mat, blanket, or block.

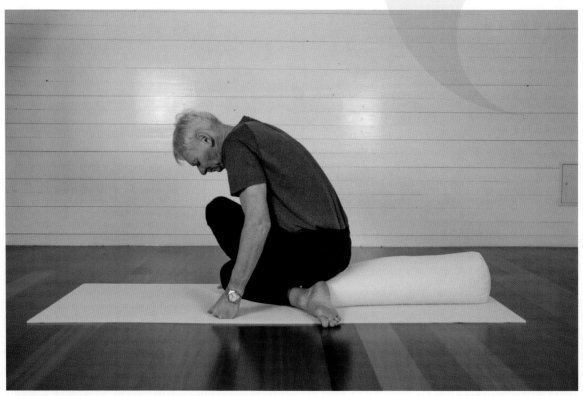

THE EASIER WAY

Problem with sitting on your bottom leg? Keep it straight and bend the top leg over. Maybe grab the bent leg to find your edge.

COUNTERPOSE

Window Wipers to bring back movement into your legs.

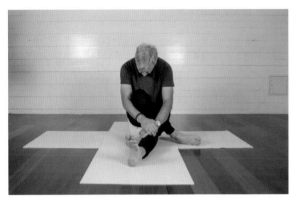

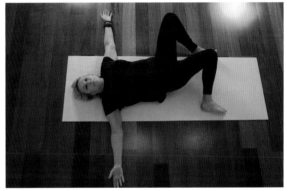

COMING OUT OF THE POSE

Let go of your top leg if you're holding it and let your legs come straight out in front of you.

TIP

Window Wipers are great on their own for increasing mobility in your hips.

Meridians

Stimulates the Liver, Kidney and Gallbladder. Bladder if you bend forward.

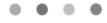

Snail

WHY IT'S GOOD FOR YOU

Snail stretches your spine—creating space between each vertebra—making you more flexible.

It can relieve backaches due to bad posture or sitting too long in front of a desk—or binge watching the TV. It also releases the shoulders, biceps, and triceps.

The physio says... Tight hamstrings draw your pelvis backward which can lead to lumbar pain. This stretch can help prevent this.

HOW TO DO IT

Lie down on your mat. Bring your legs together, arms by your sides, palms down.

Use your core to lift your hips and swing your legs up and over with your toes toward the floor.

TIP
Holding poses for time gently lengthens your fascia and mildly stresses your joints and connective tissues, increasing their range of motion.

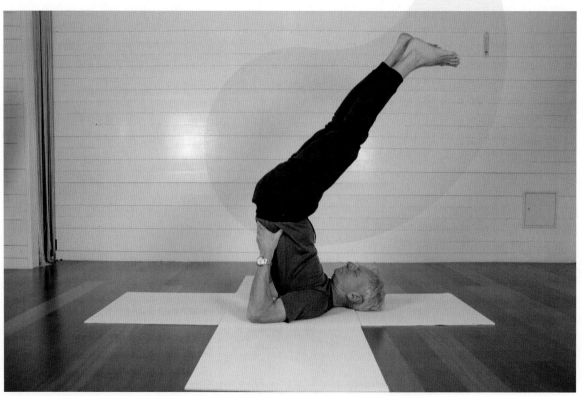

THE EASIER WAY

If like me you have tight hamstrings you can use a wall. Lie down with your head about one to two feet (thirty to sixty centimeters) away from the wall.

Now use your core to lift your hips and swing your legs up and overhead onto the wall behind you.

COUNTERPOSE

Do Window Wipers on your back or switch over onto your front and stay in Sphinx pose for a short while.

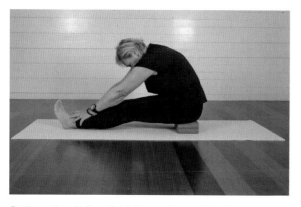

Still too hard? Just fold forward into the Caterpillar pose.

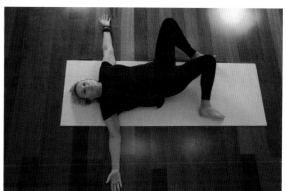

COMING OUT OF THE POSE

Roll back down until you're lying on your mat.

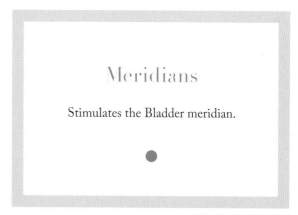

Meridians

Stimulates the Bladder meridian.

Sphinx/Seal

WHY IT'S GOOD FOR YOU

These poses help you restore your spine's natural curvature while stretching your stomach muscles and the front of your body. They also improve your nervous system by mildly stretching your hips, pelvis, and ribcage.

The physio says... We sit too much, which can lead to bulging discs. This exercise can centralize the discs, helping relieve lower back pain.

HOW TO DO IT

Starting on your stomach, use your arms to prop yourself up with your elbows beneath your shoulders.

Rest your hands on the floor or bring your palms together if you think it's more comfortable.

TIP
Focus on function, not form. How you look isn't what's important with yin yoga (or any other form of yoga). It's all about the good you are doing to your body while you're in the pose.

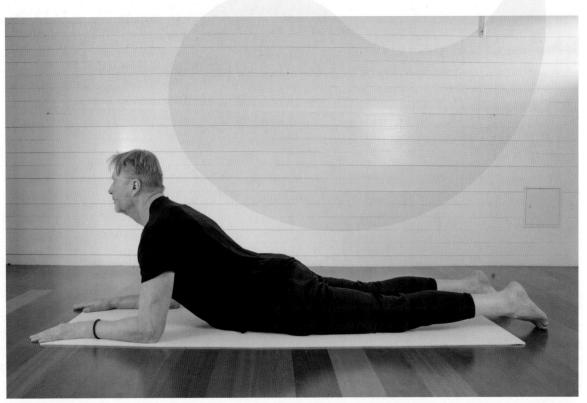

WANT MORE?

Press up from your palms to extend your arms out into Seal pose.

COUNTERPOSE

Relax into either Flapping Fish or Child's pose.

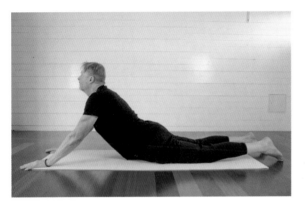

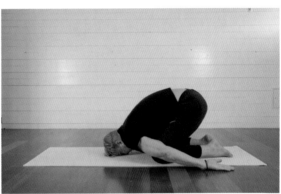

THE EASIER WAY

Maybe rest your head in your arms or on a block?

COMING OUT OF THE POSE

Lower yourself back to the ground and relax your head on either the left or right side.

Meridians

Stimulates the Kidney, Bladder, Stomach, and Spleen meridians.

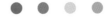

Squat

WHY IT'S GOOD FOR YOU

Squatting is our natural way to sit. It stretches our groins, hips, inner thighs, and strengthens our ankles, knees, and legs. Squatting increases flexibility and relieves stiffness and tightness.

The physio says... Try an assisted squat by holding onto something like a table. You can then find which points of your body you should concentrate on.

HOW TO DO IT

Start with your feet shoulder-width apart and squat down. Maybe push your legs apart a little with your arms?

TIP
Remember, if you're feeling pain, then back out of the pose slightly, or back out altogether and enjoy a few minutes in Savasana.

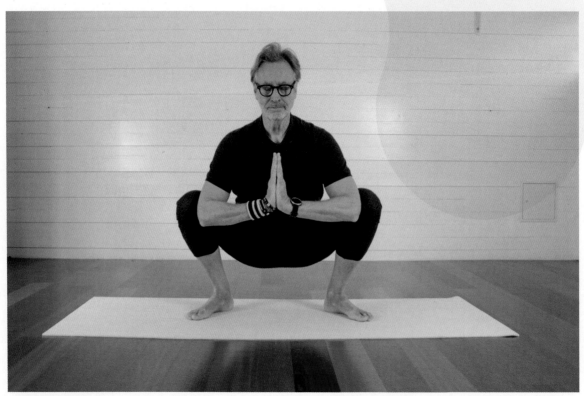

THE EASIER WAY

If you have problems squatting down—particularly under ninety degrees—grab hold of a door frame or something similar. You can also put a folded towel under your heels if they come up off the ground.

COUNTERPOSE

Try Dangling or Caterpillar for a short time.

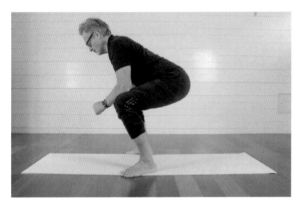

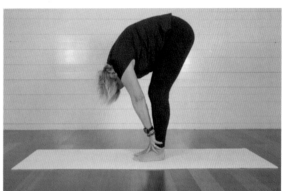

COMING OUT OF THE POSE

If you're by a door or chair, use them to pull yourself up, or simply stand up.

Meridians

Stimulates the Liver, Kidney, Bladder.
Stomach, Spleen, and Gallbladder
if you feel stretching in your ankles.

Straddle (DRAGONFLY)

WHY IT'S GOOD FOR YOU

Dragonfly increases your hip mobility and stretches your inner thighs, hamstrings, and spine as well as your abdominals. Pushing your arms out stretches the shoulders. It can lengthen the spine, making you more flexible and less prone to injury.

HOW TO DO IT

Sit with both legs straight out in front of you. Now spread your legs as far as they can go.

Make sure you tilt your hips forward, allowing your back to round which avoids too much stress. Let your hamstrings slowly fall into the mat.

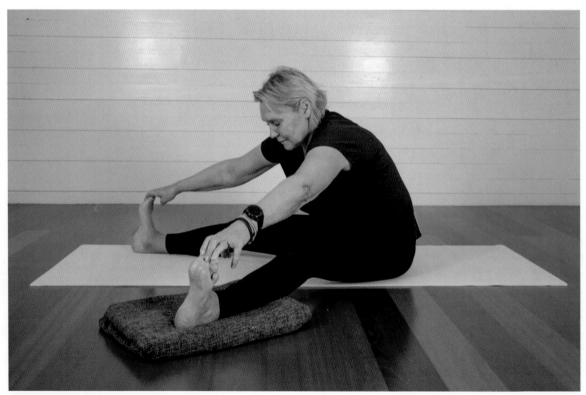

THE EASIER WAY

Sit higher on a cushion or bolster. Don't lean forward if you find it too uncomfortable at first.

COUNTERPOSE

Bring your feet together, then move them from side to side, unlocking any remaining tension.

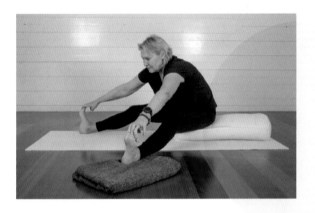

TIP
*Let gravity do the work,
not your muscles.*

COMING OUT OF THE POSE

Bring your legs back together, then use your palms to come back to a comfortable sitting position.

Meridians

Straddle stimulates the
Bladder, Liver, and Spleen meridians

● ● ●

Supine Twist/TWISTED ROOT

WHY IT'S GOOD FOR YOU

This pose stretches your back muscles and glutes, massaging your back and hips. It helps to lengthen, relax, and realign your spine while it stresses your abdominal muscles.

According to TCM, it encourages the flow of fresh blood to your digestive organs, benefitting your digestive system.

The physio says... Lots of people are tight in their chest and gluteal muscles. This pose stretches both. It's especially good for men.

HOW TO DO IT

Lie on your back with your arms out straight. Bring your legs up to your chest, then drop them to your right side.

Alternatively, keep your right leg straight, hook your left foot over your knee and use your hand to drag your left knee over to your right-hand side. Turn your head to the left (if you've come down to the right).

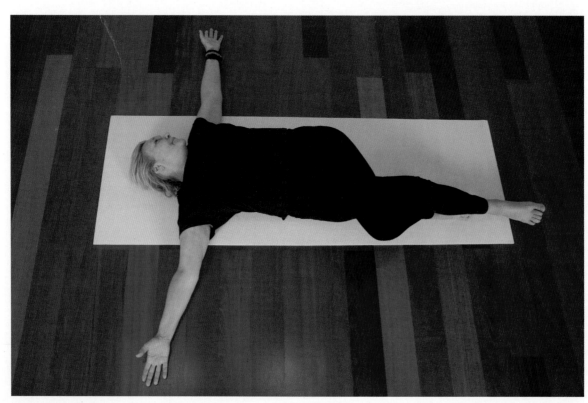

THE EASIER WAY

Rest your legs on a block or bolster.

COMING OUT OF THE POSE

Bring your knees back to the middle before dropping
them to the other side.

COUNTERPOSE

Simply do the other side.

TIP

*Once you've found your edge, push
down on your knee to increase the
stretch.*

Meridians

Stimulates the Bladder and
Gallbladder meridians.

● ●

Swan/SLEEPING SWAN

WHY IT'S GOOD FOR YOU

This is an excellent opener for your hips, legs, groin, back, knees, and ankle joints. It stretches the IT (iliotibial) band, which helps prevent knee problems.

The physio says... Try to find the spot that is tightest by moving around slightly before you settle in the pose. That way you do the best for your body – even if it's uncomfortable.

HOW TO DO IT

From Tabletop position, go into Downward Dog. Bring your right foot forward, keeping your left foot planted. Now bend your knees and sit on the floor, extending your arms in front of you and folding over your right foot. Bring your face down and rest your head in your arms or on a block.

TIP
Yin yoga is all about rest and digest. But like all sports, it's a good idea to practice on an empty stomach. Why not try early in the morning before breakfast?

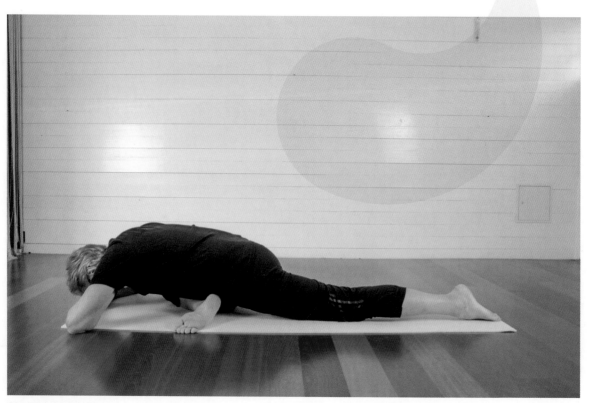

THE EASIER WAY

The Figure Four pose targets the same areas but you lie on your back, which is more comfortable.

From a lying position, bend your knees and place your feet on the floor, hip-width apart. Lift your right foot and place it over your left knee to make the

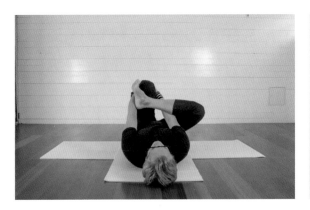

"figure of four" shape. If you wish, grab hold of your left thigh and pull it toward you for a deeper stretch.

COUNTERPOSE

You can start and finish each side in Downward Dog, which also makes an excellent counterpose.

From a Tabletop position, bring your hands in front of your shoulders, then push up through your toes until you are in an upside-down "V" pose.

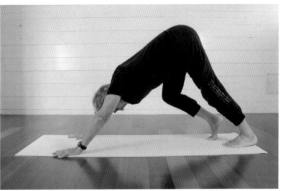

Keeping your knees slightly bent, try to push each heel down in turn so you "walk your dog."

COMING OUT OF THE POSE

Push yourself up first, then slide your bent leg backward.

Alternatively, you can push up straight into Downward Dog pose.

Meridians

Liver and Kidney, Stomach and Spleen, and Gallbladder meridians.

● ● ○ ● ○

Yin ON THE WALL

Got a wall? Then you've got all the support you need to do yin yoga. And the therapeutic benefits are the same, including reducing pain in your joints—especially the knees and hips—helping with backaches, stretching hamstrings and other muscles and connective tissues of your back and legs.

And of course, it helps you relax, relieving stress and tension overall, especially in your neck.

You can do several poses using the wall as support, including...

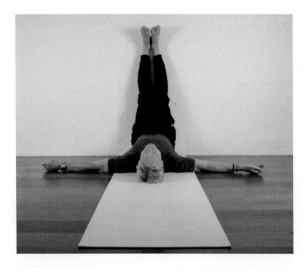

WALL CATERPILLAR

Sit sideways onto a wall, swing your legs upward, and rest onto your back. Try to wiggle closer to the wall until your sitting bones are against the wall and your legs above you.

If you find being too close to the wall uncomfortable, just move backward slightly. Have your hands either across your lap, your heart, or even out straight for a nicer back stretch. Stay for as long as it feels comfortable.

Want more support? Put a cushion under your bottom. This pose is great if your back is aching or you've been on your feet all day.

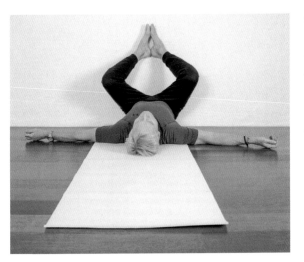

WALL BUTTERFLY

From Caterpillar, slide your legs down a bit then bring your feet together, letting your knees go as wide as the wall allows. Put your hands where they are most comfortable, over your stomach, chest, or out behind you. Stay for as long as you feel comfortable.

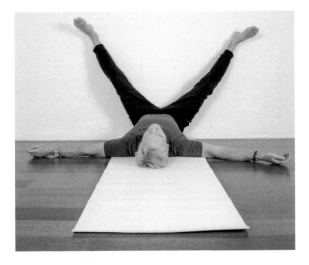

WALL STRADDLE

From Caterpillar, let your legs splay apart to the sides of the wall as deep as you can go until you find your edge. When you're ready you can use your hands to push your legs back together. Stay for as long as it feels comfortable.

WALL SQUAT

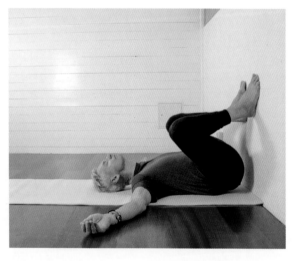

Start from Caterpillar, now bend both your knees
and slide your feet down the wall. Maybe keep them
hip-width apart. Just as in Caterpillar, if you feel it's
too hard to have your bottom right by the wall, simply
slide it away a bit. Stay for as long as it feels
comfortable.

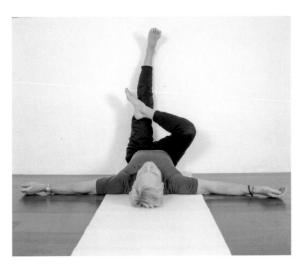

WALL FIGURE OF FOUR

Start from Caterpillar and slowly bend your straight leg, sliding your foot down the wall. Place your right ankle on your left knee. If you feel things are too tight, move away from the wall slightly.

Rest on a pillow, blanket, or bolster if you like. Stay for as long as it feels comfortable, then do the other side.

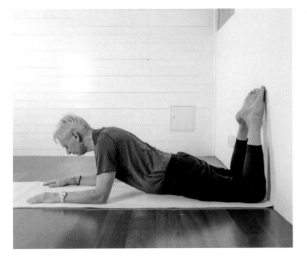

WALL SPHINX

Roll onto your stomach, bend your knees, and push yourself back to the wall. When you feel ready, push yourself up onto your elbows. Stay for as long as it feels comfortable.

Don't forget to start and finish with Savasana.

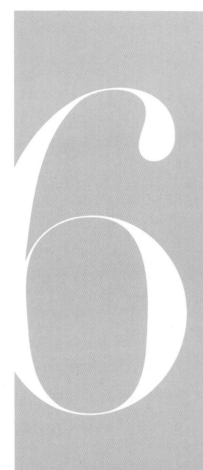

Putting the pieces together

SEQUENCES FOR A BETTER BODY
...AND MIND

The best antidote to a hectic schedule, or if you're feeling stiffness, is relaxing in yin yoga poses.

These next pages suggest yin yoga flows (sequences) to help you with everything from headaches to hamstrings and stimulate your body from the tops of your fingers to the tips of your toes.

While most of the sequences below concentrate on helping with specific body issues, others help you perform better in sports such as golf, skiing, and hiking, or just help to make everyday life that much easier, meaning that carrying shopping or humping around grandkids becomes less of a chore.

All sequences start and end with Savasana, Corpse pose. I feel that it gives us the opportunity to scan our bodies both before and after the practice.

Take the time to make the time

These flows are all between fifty to seventy minutes long, which you may feel is too long if you're not at a class.

Do what feels right for you. If you only have time for a few of the poses, fine. It's a lot better than none. You can even check out the fifteen-minute fixes further in the book.

Let's do it.

Introduction to yin yoga sequence

This introductory flow gives you a nice, whole-body massage. It's a perfect start to your yin yoga exploration, and hopefully will spur you on to trying all the flows in this section.

Start by lying in Savasana, Corpse pose. Relax with your palms up and breathe. Feel your weight, soften your jaw and sense through your body.

After a few minutes, put your right hand onto your heart and your left hand onto your belly button. As you breathe in deeply, extend your belly button until it is above your heart. Now breathe out slowly. Try this for eight to ten breaths.

Pose 1: RECLINING BUTTERFLY

Three minutes
This is a nice pose that takes the pressure off your hips and knees, reducing the chance of chronic pain in those areas.

To come out of the pose, bring your hands down by your sides then push your knees together, using your hands if you need to. Rest in this position before you try the counterpose.

Counterpose: Teepee or Window Wipers.

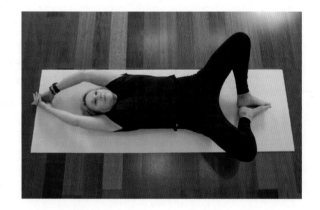

Pose 2: SPHINX/SEAL

Three minutes
Restore the natural curvature of your spine and keep your lower back healthy with this gentle stretch.

To come out of the pose, simply lie back down. Enjoy a rest with your head on one side before you do a counterpose.

Counterpose: Flapping Fish/Child's pose. Stay in either of these poses for a few minutes to enjoy the stretch.

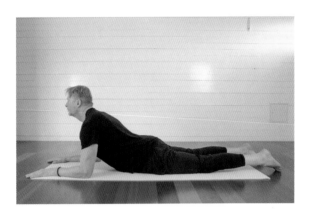

Pose 3: CATERPILLAR

Four minutes
This excellent hamstring stretch is also good for stimulating the deeper tendons and the tissues around your spine and abdominals.

If you feel that this pose is a bit too much for you, lie on your back with your legs up a wall.

To come out of the pose, use your hands to push yourself up.

Counterpose: Lean back and move your feet from side to side to loosen up your hips, or do Window Wipers. Try for ten on each side.

Remember. Let gravity do the work, not your muscles.

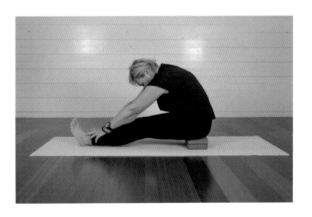

Pose 4: DRAGON

Three minutes each side
A great hip and groin opener, Dragon poses help target your hip flexors and quads in your back leg.

When you're ready, push back with your hands, or come into Downward Dog.

Counterpose: Move your spine gently backward and forward from Tabletop.

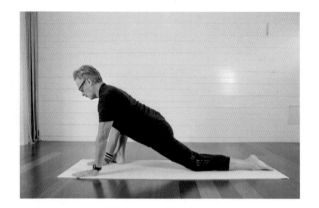

Pose 5: SUPINE TWIST / TWISTED ROOT

Three minutes
A great tension releaser for your spine, lower back, and neck. It stretches the obliques, glutes, hips, and IT band.

Counterpose: Do the other side.

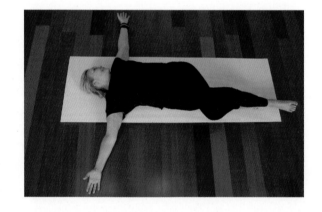

Ending. *Savasana for five minutes or as long as you like*

How does your body feel now? Scan it. Feel it. Relax into the mat.

Coming out
Stretch, curl. Come up very slowly.

ASYMMETRIC POSES FOR
a more symmetrical body

As we age, our bodies become more asymmetrical, putting pressure on one side more than the other. The result is that we can end up with shoulder, back, hip, knee, and ankle problems on the side that is most tense and where muscles, tendons, and ligaments are shorter.

This sequence of asymmetrical poses (stretching each side independently) is designed to bring back some of the symmetry we may have lost over the years.

Beginning. *Savasana*

Do a guided body scan. Go through your body from your neck, through your shoulders, biceps, hips, knees, calves, and ankles. How are they feeling?

Feel your weight, soften your jaw. Check out each side of your body.

Try some 4x4 breathing in and out to relax your body and mind.

Pose 1: B A N A N A S A N A

Three minutes each side
This side bend stretches your muscles from the IT band to the intercostal muscles in the ribcage, your stomach muscles and even your biceps and triceps.

Counterpose: Hug/circle your knees.

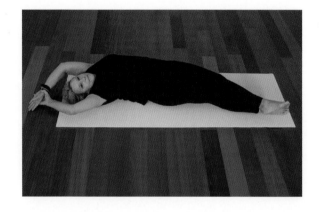

Pose 2: HALF BUTTERFLY

Three minutes each side
This "best of both worlds" pose stretches your lower back and is great for tight hamstrings. It targets the ligaments along the back of the spine as well as the adductor (groin) muscles on your bent leg, opening up your hip.

Counterpose: Teepee, Window Wipers.

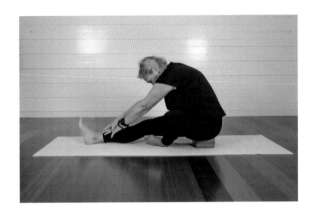

Pose 3: DRAGON

Three minutes each side
A super hip and groin opener that also stretches your glutes, hip flexors, and quads in your stretched leg.

Counterpose: Gently rock backward and forward in Tabletop.

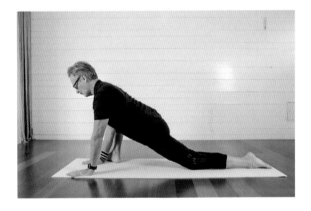

Pose 4: SLEEPING SWAN

Three minutes each side

Sleeping Swan targets your front leg, stretching your quads and hip flexors, as well as your IT band. It stretches your ankles on your extended leg.

Counterpose: Downward Dog or Child's pose.

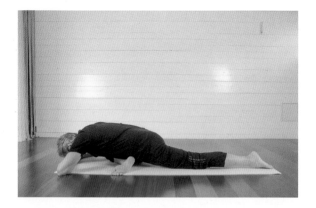

Pose 5: SUPINE TWIST /TWISTED ROOT

Three minutes each side

This pose is great for releasing tension in your upper spine while stretching your shoulder joint. If you suffer from sciatica, then bring your bent knee closer to your chest to see if it helps.

Counterpose: Do the other side.

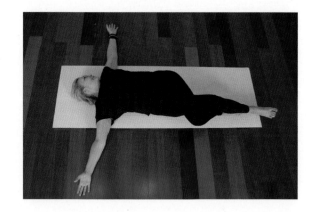

Ending. *Savasana for five minutes*

How's the left side of your body now compared to the right side?

We talk about bringing the symmetry back to our bodies. So that maybe means working on areas that are tightest, rather than working exactly three minutes per side? The more symmetric we become, the less likely we are to suffer from the pain of overexerting one side. It's obvious if you think about it.

A sequence for aching
SHOULDERS AND SPINE

Many people have problems with their shoulders, spine, and necks as they get older. If we don't stretch these areas, they stiffen, become inflamed and arthritic, and could lead to us having to have an operation—if we haven't had one already.

This flow helps us free up our shoulders and spines, hopefully preventing these problems.

Beginning. *Savasana for four minutes*

Feel your weight. Soften your jaw. Sense through your body. Scan from the top, through your neck, shoulders, back, vertebrae, around the hips, and the base of your spine.

Practice box breathing (4x4 breathing). Try to go from all the outside impulses to what's happening inside your body, your mind, your psyche.

Pose 1: MELTING HEART

Three minutes
This is a great pose for opening your shoulders and back, as well as stretching out your arms. It releases pressure in your chest and loosens the muscles in your middle and lower back.

Counterpose: Lie in Flapping Fish pose and stretch each arm for a minute or so when you come out of the pose.

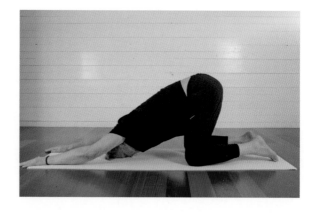

Pose 2: OPEN WING

Three minutes each side

I really like this pose as it helps push my shoulders back and relieves tension along my arm. It also helps me with tennis elbow by stretching the tendons of my lower arm.

Counterpose: Thread the Needle. Bring your arm down and through the supporting arm.

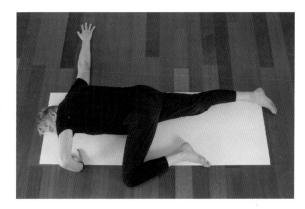

Pose 3: SPHINX/SEAL

Three to four minutes

This is a great way to help keep your lower back more supple. Keeping your lower back healthy will affect the rest of your spine and helps improve your posture, so that you don't start leaning forward with your head bent toward the floor.

You're also stretching your stomach muscles. Six pack at 60 anyone?

Don't fancy Sphinx or Seal? Do Supported Bridge.

Counterpose: Flapping Fish/Child's pose.

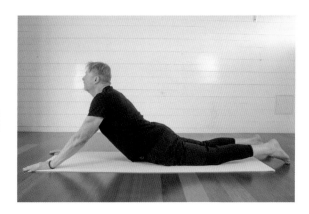

Pose 4: RECLINING BUTTERFLY

Four minutes each side
This pose targets the ligaments along the back of your spine when you're lying down.

A good idea is to support yourself with a block or blanket. If your bones feel supported, your muscles relax.

Counterpose: Teepee/Window Wipers are great counterposes.

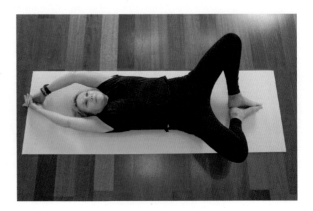

Pose 5: DRAGONFLY

Three minutes
Because you're leaning forward as well as separating your legs, this pose is great for increasing spine and hip mobility.

Try to separate your legs as far as your edge allows. If you wish, you can sit upright and pull the left side of your head with your right hand and vice versa to loosen your neck and the top of your shoulders.

Counterpose: Lean back onto your elbows, keep your legs straight and wiggle your feet from side to side.

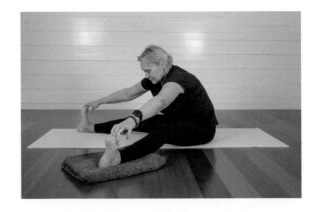

Pose 6: SUPINE TWIST
/TWISTED ROOT

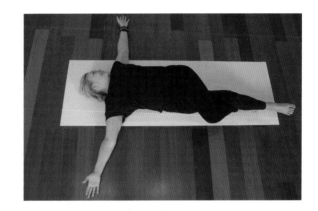

Three minutes each side
A lovely stretch to lengthen, relax, and realign your
spine. Keep your shoulders flat on the floor to
stimulate the muscles at the front of your chest,
relieving tension in your shoulders.

Counterpose: Do the other side.

Ending. *Savasana for five minutes*

While you're relaxing in Savasana, think about being
more mindful. The three ideas behind mindfulness are:

1. **Live in the moment.** Try to be open and
accepting. Find joy in what's simple.

2. **Accept yourself.** Treat yourself the way you
would treat a good friend.

3. **Focus on your breath** as it moves in and out
of your body.

A sequence for relieving
STIFF BACKS AND SCIATICA

The most common form of back pain is when you sit or lift things incorrectly, creating what's called postural stress.

When we sit down—which we do for long hours, in front of computer screens or watching streaming channels—we cause our backs to curve. According to the Cornell University Department of Ergonomics, we add close to ninety percent as much pressure to our discs when we're sitting than when we're standing.

WHAT IS SCIATICA?

Sciatica is the pain that results from irritation or inflammation of the sciatic nerve as it winds its way from your lumbar spine down through your legs. It frequently flares up while bending over, running, sitting (especially driving), and during other active or passive everyday movements.

WHAT CAUSES SCIATICA?

The medical community agrees that the most common cause of sciatica comes from the spine where disc problems can create direct pressure on the roots of your sciatic nerve.

Another cause is piriformis syndrome where the piriformis muscle has become shortened, pressing down on the sciatic nerve. The piriformis is a flat, narrow muscle that runs from your spine through your bottom to the top of your thighs.

Beginning. *Savasana for four minutes*

If you want a variation on Savasana you can try Pentacle pose where you move your arms so that they are square to your body, and space out your legs by putting your feet on the sides of your mat.

Savasana relaxes your body and can improve your posture, helping to relieve sciatica.

Pose 1: CATERPILLAR

Three minutes

Caterpillar relieves pressure on your lower back and sciatic nerve. It also relieves back pain by rotating your pelvis slightly.

Counterpose: Hug your knees to your chest.

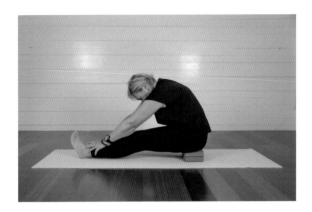

Pose 2: WIDE-KNEE CHILD'S POSE

Four minutes

Child's pose helps stretch your spine, making your lower back, hips, and thighs more flexible, while stretching the muscles around the nerve.

Counterpose: Cat/cow.

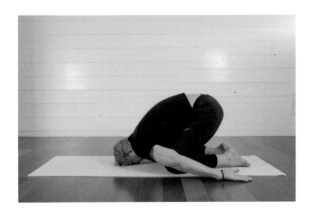

Pose 3: SLEEPING SWAN OR FIGURE OF FOUR

Four minutes each side
This stretch can help relieve sciatica by externally rotating your front leg, stretching your quads, hip flexors, IT band, and piriformis muscle.

Counterpose: Downward Dog.

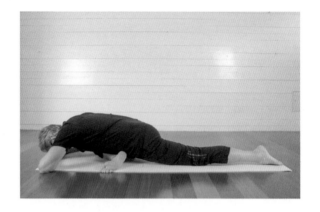

Pose 4: HALF/FULL SHOELACE

Two minutes each side or four minutes
Shoelace helps decompress your lower back and relieves pressure on your sciatic nerve.

Counterpose: Deer pose.

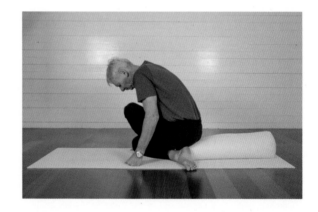

Pose 5: DRAGONFLY

Four minutes
Short hamstrings stress your lower back and can cause or aggravate back pain and sciatica. This pose stretches your hamstrings and inner thighs to increase hip mobility, which should help relieve back pain.

Counterpose: Window Wipers.

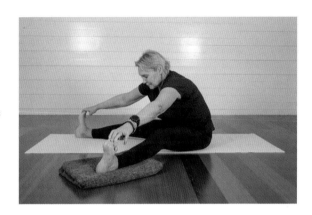

Ending. *Savasana for five minutes*

Enjoy five minutes of relaxation for a deep rest that releases the tension—and pain—in your body. Try supporting your knees and/or your lower back with a blanket or bolster to increase relaxation and decrease pressure on your back and nervous system.

How does your back feel now?

A sequence for golfers

Are the fairways getting longer as you get older? Are you getting that back twinge from hole 14 onward? Try this sequence especially for golfers. It irons out stiffness and brings the spring back to your driver, and your body.

Choose from the exercises below to improve your golf—and your score.

Beginning. *Savasana for four minutes*

Try to keep your eyes closed. Relax. Breathe deeply to release your fascia.

Pose 1: RECLINING BUTTERFLY

Three minutes
Reclining Butterfly is an excellent pose to stretch your lower back and increase pelvic rotation for your downswing as well as your setup by having your arms stretched out.

Counterpose: Teepee or Window Wipers.

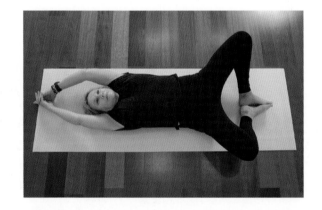

Pose 2: MELTING HEART

Three minutes
This pose opens your shoulders and upper back, stretching your arms. It benefits the takeaway and the downswing.

Counterpose: Child's pose.

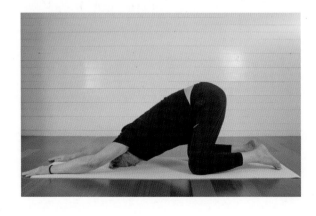

Pose 3: OPEN WING

Three minutes each side
Open Wing targets the deeper tissues of the shoulders, releasing tensions, even in the hips. It's ideal for all aspects of your golf swing.

Counterpose: Bring your right arm through in the opposite direction. Threading the Needle.

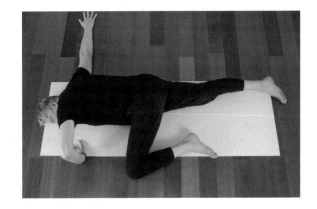

Pose 4: SPHINX/SEAL

Three minutes
These poses improve posture while you stretch the front of your torso and your stomach muscles, helping with rotation throughout your swing.

Counterpose: Flapping Fish.

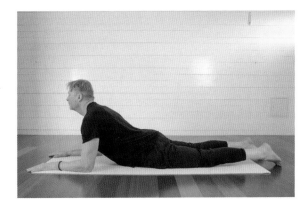

Pose 5: DRAGON

Three minutes each side
Dragon poses target your hip flexors and quads, helping you move better through impact, so you can drive the ball harder.

Counterpose: Moving back and forward from Tabletop.

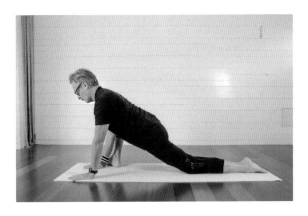

Pose 6: DRAGONFLY

Three minutes
Dragonfly increases your hip mobility, helping you set up the right posture and maintain it through your swing.

Counterpose: Lean back and move your feet from side to side.

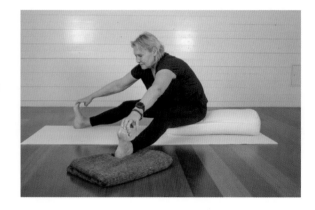

Pose 7: SWAN/SLEEPING SWAN

Three minutes per side. Or figure of 4.
By externally rotating your front leg you release pressure on your knees and hips, helping you rotate through your golf swing.

Counterpose: Downward Dog.

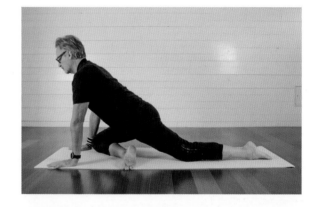

Pose 8: RECLINING TWIST

Three minutes per side
The separation between hips and torso during this stretch is perfect for adding those extra yards to your shot.

Counterpose: Do the other side.

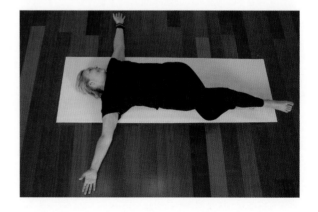

Ending. *Savasana as long as you like*

How's the left side, how's the right side?

We talk about bringing the symmetry back to our bodies. More symmetry means less pain and more pleasure on the golf course, as your hips, back, legs, shoulders, and knees should be more aligned. Swing on.

A sequence for walkers and hikers

Like to hike but your legs are starting to protest? As we age, our lower bodies tighten up the most. We lose mobility from the navel down.

When we practice yin yoga we stimulate the growth of fibroblasts. These are the cells responsible for creating collagen, elastin, and the molecules that hydrate our joints and tissues. Hydrating our tissues allows our joints to move and our fascia to slide more easily. The result is that we feel less stiff, and enjoy walking much more.

This sequence targets your quads, inner thighs, hamstrings, hip flexors, and hip joints to keep you moving along the trail for longer, and without feeling so stiff.

Remember. If you feel any pain in any pose, back off or come out of the pose directly.

Beginning. *Savasana for five minutes*

Try some belly breathing. Lift your belly in as you inhale. Do a quick body scan and try to make your spine as long as possible.

Pose 1: BUTTERFLY

Four minutes
Butterfly stretches your inner thighs, groins, knees, and hamstrings. It also targets your ligaments along the back of the spine, keeping you comfortable on your feet for longer.

Counterpose: Lean back with your feet together and wave them from side to side.

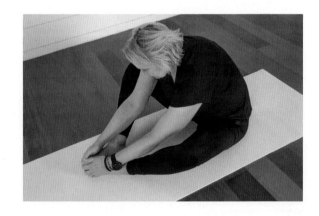

Pose 2: DRAGONFLY (STRADDLE)

Three minutes
This pose helps with hip mobility and stretches your inner thighs, hamstrings, spine, and abdominals. It makes walking more comfortable… or life more comfortable after walking.

Counterpose: From a leaning back position, move your feet from side to side.

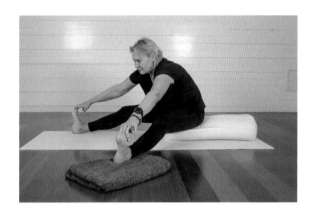

Pose 3: SLEEPING SWAN /FIGURE OF FOUR

Four minutes each side
This pose stresses your IT band, helping relieve knee and hip problems, increasing your hiking pleasure.

Counterpose: Downward Dog.

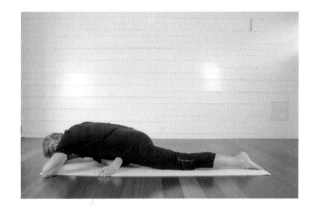

Pose 4: SHOELACE

Three minutes each side
Shoelace stretches your inner thighs and groin as well as loosening your hips. Looser hips means easier walking.

Counterpose: Teepee or Window Wipers.

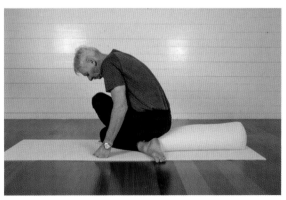

Pose 5: SADDLE

Three minutes each side
I find this a tough one but get lots of benefit from it as it gives my hip flexors and quadriceps a really good stretch. It's excellent for people who do a lot of standing or walking.

Counterpose: Relax in Savasana for a short time before pulling your knees to your chest, maybe one at a time, to release your lower back.

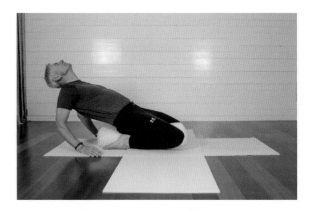

Pose 6: BANANASANA

Three minutes per side
Stretching all of one side then the other takes tension off the whole side including your legs. It's perfect before or after a long hike.

Counterpose: Hug/circle your knees.

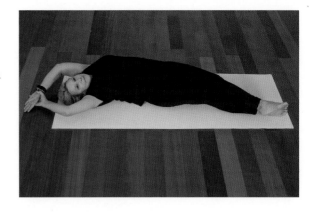

Ending. *Savasana as long as you like*

Check out how your body feels now. Hopefully you should feel a lot less leggy.

A sequence for better sleep

There's nothing like a good night's sleep to feel better throughout the day. Your body rests and repairs itself, while you boost your immune system and help prevent diseases. And it's good for warding off depression and improving your memory.

But if you forgot the last time you slept for as long as you need to, try this flow to send you into the land of dreams. You don't need to do every pose, just the ones you think will help you sleep.

Beginning. *Savasana for four minutes*

This slow start to any yin yoga session helps you calm your body and brings back its natural balance. Practice Ocean breath while you relax ever deeper.

Pose 1: CHILD'S POSE

Three minutes
Child's pose is the perfect way to relax and soothe your mind, all while you give your spine a lovely stretch.

Counterpose: Tabletop.

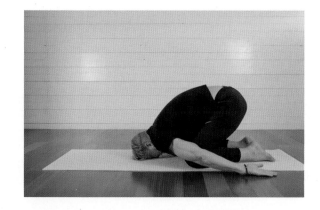

Pose 2: FROG POSE

Three minutes
This excellent hip opener helps stretch your inner thighs and improves range of motion as well as helping relieve lower back tension. That should help you sleep better.

Counterpose: Lie on your back and pull your knees to your chest.

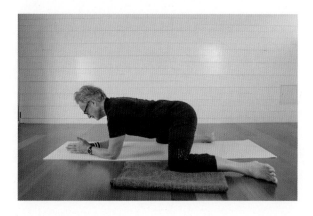

Pose 3: SUPPORTED BRIDGE

Three minutes
Supported bridge helps relieve headaches, soothes
your nervous system, and promotes relaxation. Use
props like bolsters and blankets to support your hips,
knees, and feet if you want.

Counterpose: Hug your knees to your chest.

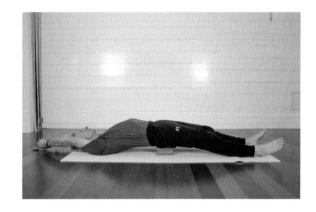

Pose 4: DEER POSE

Three minutes each side
This restful hip opening pose is excellent for relieving
stress and tension in your hips and lower back. Why
not rest onto a bolster and dream away?

Counterpose: Window Wipers.

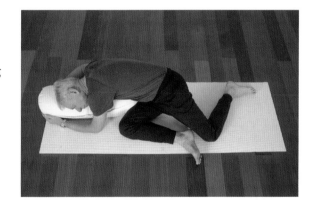

Pose 5: HAPPY BABY

Three minutes
Happy Baby helps reduce back pain and can ease any
stress or anxiety you may be feeling. Like all yin yoga
poses, it lowers your heart rate, making sleep easier.

Counterpose: Child's pose.

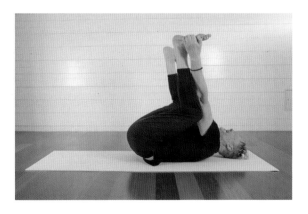

Pose 6: WALL CATERPILLAR

Three minutes

Wall Caterpillar is the perfect antidote to a long day on your feet. It's an excellent pose for calming your body and making you less anxious; super-important for a good night's sleep.

Counterpose: Drop right into Wall Butterfly.

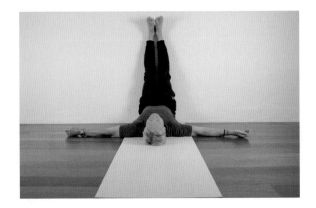

Pose 7: WALL BUTTERFLY

Three minutes

Enjoy relaxing by the wall. Having your legs in Butterfly, yet above your head while you control your breathing is a great way to slow your body and mind.

Both these wall poses on their own are a great way to get ready for bed. Use props to make yourself as comfortable as you can.

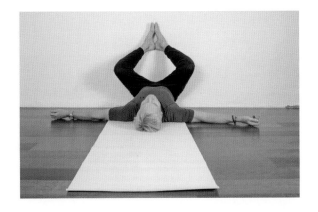

Pose 8: S U P I N E   T W I S T

Three minutes each side
Enjoy this gentle twisting motion of your spine as it
relieves the tension in your back.

Counterpose: Do the other side.

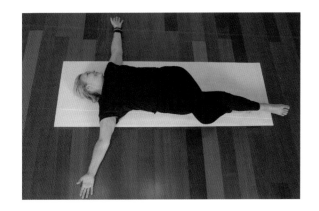

Ending. *Savasana for five minutes*

Use deep breathing in this pose to really let go of your
worries. Concentrate inward on yourself, your body,
and your mind.

Now enjoy that glass of herbal tea before you get that
good night's rest.

A sequence for HEALTHIER KNEES AND HIPS

A lifetime of using our knees and hips means that they've taken a lot of stress and could be on the way to wearing out—if they haven't done already.

This sequence helps bring that little bit of flexibility back to our most important tissues when it comes to mobility, so you can keep on rocking—even if you've already got an artificial joint or two.

Beginning. *Savasana for four minutes*

Enjoy some peace before you start the sequence. Think about your hips and knees in particular. Is there any one area that is stiffer than the other? In my case, I feel the outside of my left knee, but when I concentrate I understand that I have a tight left groin. Releasing the groin takes the pressure off my knee.

Pose 1: BUTTERFLY

Three minutes
Butterfly stretches the knee and thigh muscles, promoting movement and relieving pain

Counterpose: Deer pose.

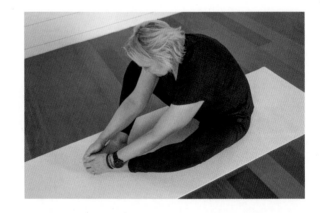

Pose 2: SPHINX/SEAL

Three minutes
These poses increase range of motion in your joints, relieving pressure and pain from your hips and knees. Be careful if you have a problem with your back. Find your edge and don't push it.

Counterpose: Child's pose.

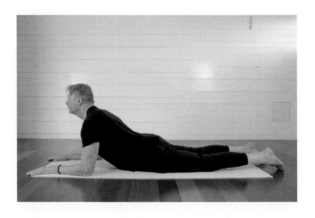

Pose 3: S Q U A T

As long as you feel comfortable
This is an excellent way to relieve pressure on our hips, ankles, and knees. If you find squatting a problem, hold on to a table leg or a staircase.

Counterpose: Dangling.

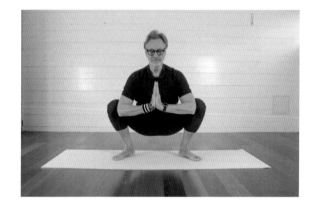

Pose 4: S L E E P I N G   S W A N

Three minutes each side
Extending your hip flexors and stretching your IT band relieves pressure on these important muscles and joints. For extra comfort, rest your bottom or the side of your bent leg on a bolster.

Counterpose: Downward Dog.

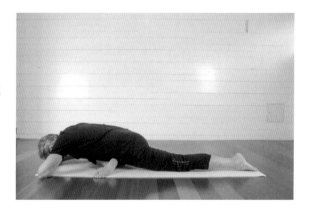

Pose 5: HALF SADDLE

Three minutes each side

This is a great way to stretch your hip flexors and quads, relieving tension in all your lower joints.

Counterpose: Supine twist for three minutes each side.

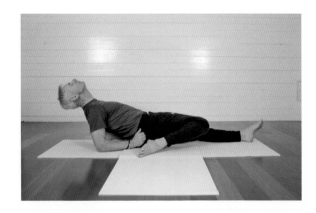

Pose 6: SUPINE TWIST

Three minutes each side

This excellent hip rotation pose stretches the tendons to the knee on your outside leg as well as freeing up your hip. Make it feel restorative by resting your knees on a bolster. Try putting a cushion or block between your knees for even more relaxation in the pose.

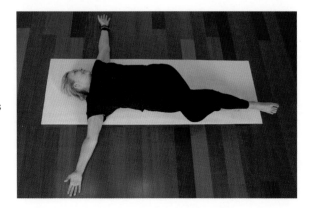

Ending. *Savasana as long as you like*

Savasana relaxes the tissues around your hips and knees.
Five minutes or more will help release stress and make you feel less tired.

A 30-minute sequence
FOR IMPROVING DIGESTION

You might be wondering if your headache, bloated stomach, and/or acid reflux is because of your diet. The chances are it is, especially as our bodies take longer to process what we ingest as we get older.

Certain yin yoga poses can help with stomach issues by relieving stress as they stimulate your rest and digest system.

Any pose that stretches or twists the abdominal muscles can regulate digestion as you're giving your stomach and intestines a gentle massage.

Beginning. *Savasana for five minutes*

This pose lowers the tempo of your mind and body before you start. You shift from a sympathetic state to a parasympathetic state.

Pose 1: SUPPORTED BRIDGE

Four minutes
This is a great way to stretch your abdominal muscles. It helps stimulate the thyroid gland which can improve your metabolism.

Counterpose: Hug your knees to your chest for two minutes.

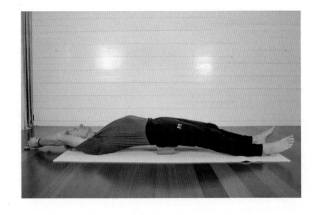

Pose 2: SQUAT

Two to three minutes
While squatting may be challenging, it pushes blood through your body a bit quicker, improving circulation and helping with the passage of food.

Counterpose: Dangling. A perfect counterpose to the squat as it stretches your hamstrings and hips. As you come out of Dangling you stimulate fresh blood, nutrients, and oxygen, improving digestion and boosting your metabolism.

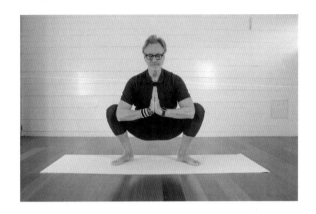

Pose 3: RECLINING TWIST

Three minutes each side
This is the perfect pose to untie any knots you may have in your stomach, relaxing your abdomen, and letting food pass through. It's a nice way to relax your stomach before you go to bed.

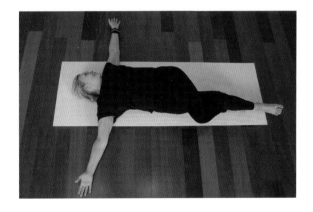

Pose 4: CHILD'S POSE

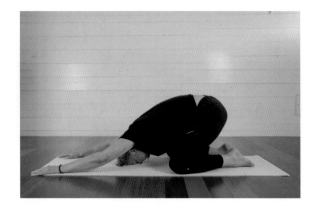

Three minutes
Another great pose to help you relax and let your intestines do what they need to do.

Counterpose: Cat/Cow.

Ending. *Savasana for five minutes*

Lie down, relax, and feel the benefit you've just given to your stomach. Enjoy the rest of your day—or a good night's sleep now there's less chance of your stomach interrupting.

A sequence for skiers

Still enjoy swooshing down slopes and cutting those carve turns in newly-pisted snow? The gentle stretching and strengthening of yin yoga is your way to prolong your skiing for years to come.

This flow concentrates on your knees, ankles, and hips, getting you in condition for whatever piste or weather conditions you encounter. Try some or all of these poses depending on how you're feeling either before or after you hit the slopes, or both!

Bring on the snow.

Beginning. *Savasana for five minutes*

Think about whether you have any specific problems with your knees, ankles, or hips, and work out if you need to spend more time on one side or the other.

Pose 1: ANKLE STRETCH

One to three minutes
This pose strengthens your ankles, keeping your feet healthy in your ski boots.
OK, so your ankles are often stuck in your boots, but the more flexible they are, the better you can steer and edge your skis, and the more fun you'll get from a day on the slopes.

Counterpose: Downward Dog.

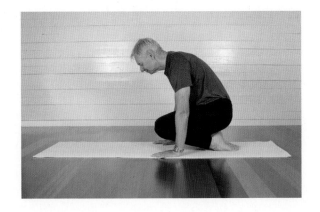

Pose 2: DRAGON POSE

Three minutes per leg
Whichever Dragon you try will stretch your hip flexors, making you more mobile on the moguls. Your hip flexors give you the ability to drive down slopes and absorb the forces on your body while taking the pressure off your lower back.

Counterpose: Child's pose. Great for skiers as it stretches your lower back, which is particularly at risk when skiing. Also good for stretching the quads that get a hammering after a day on the piste.

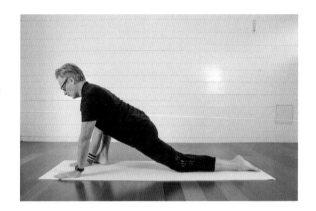

Pose 3: RECLINING BUTTERFLY

Three minutes
This pose stretches your lower back and your hip flexors, so important when you're skiing all day long—or even until lunchtime.

Counterpose: Window Wipers. An excellent way to get the right movement in your legs and hips for carving.

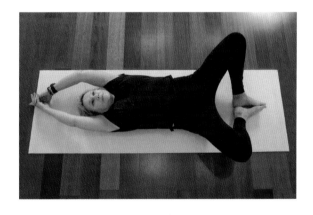

Pose 4: DANGLING

Three minutes
Doing this pose helps loosen your hamstrings, and stretch your spine and calves. All the things you need for the perfect piste performance.

Counterpose: Squat as far as you can for a minute or so to put pressure on your Achilles tendons, stretch your back, and open your hips.

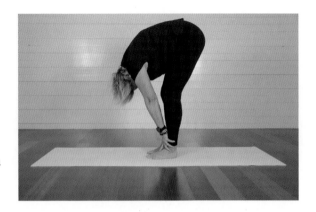

Ending. *Savasana as long as you like*

Like other sports, don't think, do. Trust yourself and your technique and maybe simply count your turns to enjoy the slopes and ski them better.

15-minute fixes to

GET YOU READY FOR ANYTHING

Got fifteen minutes? Of course you have. And while a longer yin yoga stretch would do wonders for both your physical and mental wellbeing, just fifteen minutes a day concentrating on a specific area of your body will make a huge difference to how you feel (and probably how you look).

Regular stretching—in this case through yin yoga poses—helps your body to relax, improves your range of motion, boosts your heart health, and staves off some of the effects of aging.

A FIFTEEN-MINUTE FIX to start your day

You've seen how a cat stretches when it wakes up, so why shouldn't you do the same? This short flow gets you ready for the day, and you don't even need to get out of bed to do it.

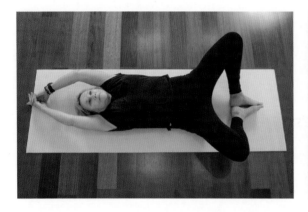

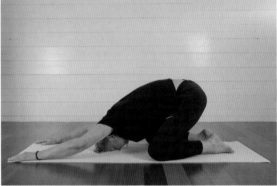

Pose 1: RECLINING BUTTERFLY

Hands by your sides or behind your head for two to three minutes
You're bound to be feeling tight when you wake up. So just couple your hands behind your head, drag your feet up so they are flat, then put the soles of your feet together and let your legs flop. After a while you'll feel the benefit in your hips.

After a couple of minutes, uncouple your hands and use your palms to push your knees together. Stay like this for a few seconds up to a minute.

Pose 2: CHILD'S POSE

Three minutes
This is a lovely way to get that cat-like stretch into your lower back, your knees, hips, and ankles.

Flip onto your stomach then come up onto your knees and palms before pushing your hips back. Keep your knees apart and your feet together. Now breathe and enjoy.

When you've finished, lie down onto your back.

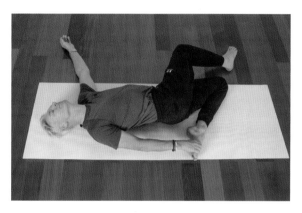

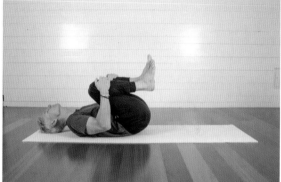

Pose 3: CAT PULLING ITS TAIL

Two minutes each side

Now let's pull a bit at our hip flexors to wake them up. You might want to prop yourself up on your right elbow. Slide your left leg over your right leg, then grab hold of your right foot.

Pull your foot until you feel the stretch in the top of your hips.

After a couple of minutes let go and pull the other foot. Roll onto your back when you've finished.

Pose 4: PULL YOUR KNEES TO YOUR STOMACH

Three minutes

As the name says, just grab hold of your knees and pull them to your chest. If you want, you can pull one leg at a time into your chest to give your stomach muscles a workout before you get out of bed.

Savasana

Three minutes

Once you've released your knees, relax back into Savasana, and concentrate on deep breathing to help you relax before you get out of bed.

Now pop into the kitchen and put the kettle on.

A FIFTEEN-MINUTE FIX FOR office bound shoulders

Hunching over a screen or glaring at a TV sitting in the wrong way can be a pain. Literally. This fifteen-minute shoulder fix will help you loosen your neck and shoulder blades, and even give you a better posture, both at work and at rest.

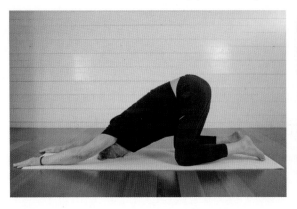

Pose 1: MELTING HEART

Three minutes
Melting Heart is the perfect upper and middle-shoulder opener. Use a blanket to rest your forehead on to be more comfortable. If you want a deeper stretch, rest on your chin (which some people find uncomfortable) or stretch your arms over a bolster.

Pose 2: OPEN WING

Two minutes each side
If your shoulders are really tight, just concentrate on using your hand to exert pressure on your extended arm. If you want more, bring your top arm all the way over.

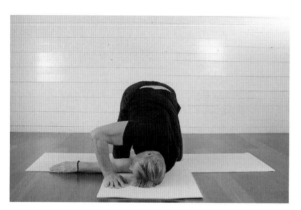

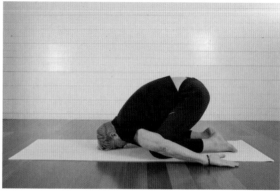

Pose 3: THREAD THE NEEDLE

Two minutes each side
This is a nice way to wake up your shoulders, upper
back and neck, helping improve your range of motion.
Relieving tension in your shoulders helps you unwind
after a busy day.

Pose 4: CHILD'S POSE

Three minutes
Child's pose helps you relax while you stretch your
spine and shoulders, hips and ankles. Concentrate on
your breathing to bring that little extra harmony to
your body—and freedom to your shoulders.

A FIFTEEN-MINUTE FIX TO
boost your back

Ouch. Your back just keeps on hurting.

Try this quick session to unlock stiff vertebrae and unleash some much-needed energy.

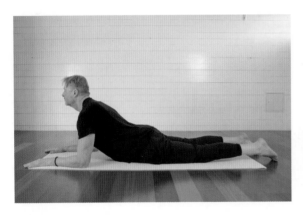

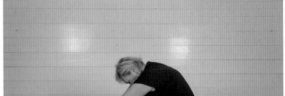

Pose 1: SPHINX

Three minutes
This pose is good for releasing tension in the small of your back and realigning your natural posture. If you feel the pose is a bit too tight, maybe spread your legs apart slightly.

Once you're done, relax on your stomach for a while and enjoy some stillness.

Pose 2: CATERPILLAR

Three minutes
Lots of people have short hamstrings, which stress your back by pulling on your sitting bones. Caterpillar stresses the ligaments along your spine, which can relieve back pain.

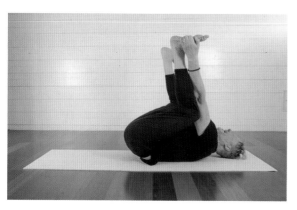

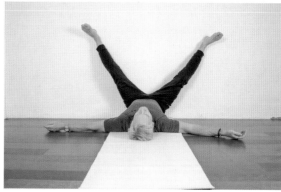

Pose 3: HAPPY BABY

Three minutes

A lovely pose to release tightness in your spine and to help realign it by lengthening and opening your lower back.

Don't worry if you can't grab hold of your feet. Grabbing your ankles or shins works too.

When you come out of Happy Baby, stretch your whole body as long as you can, from the tips of your toes to the tops of your fingers.

Pose 4: WALL STRADDLE

Four minutes

A nice, relaxing way to lengthen and stretch your back muscles as well as your hamstrings. And of course, the closer you can shimmy up to the wall, the deeper the stretch.

A FIFTEEN-MINUTE FIX TO
protect your piriformis

Wondering what your piriformis is? It's a small muscle in your buttocks behind your gluteus maximus (not a Roman general). Your piriformis can become inflamed from injury, overuse through too much exercise such as walking, or tightening or swelling. It's a pain in the bum. Literally.

This fifteen-minute fix aims to stretch the area around your piriformis and improve your range of motion.

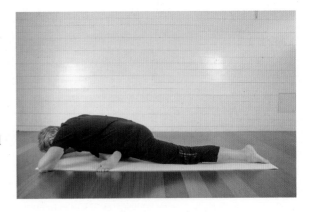

Pose 1: SLEEPING SWAN

Three minutes each side
A nice stretch for your gluteal muscles and inner thighs to relieve tightness. Maybe stretch out in Downward Dog for a while when you come out?

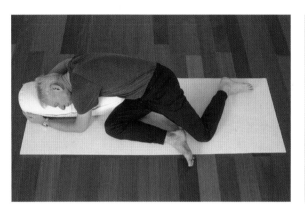

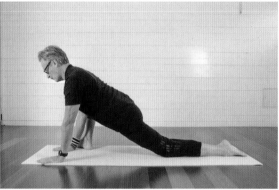

Pose 2: DEER POSE

Three minutes each side
If you've been sitting for too long, then Deer pose is an excellent stretch for your lower back, gluteal muscles, hips, and quads. Lie on a bolster to really enjoy being in the pose.

Pose 3: INSIDE DRAGON

Two minutes each side
This is a lovely way to open up your hip flexors and quads. It takes the strain from the front side of your body and relieves tension on your lower back.

A FIFTEEN-MINUTE FIX FOR *healthier hips*

Hips don't lie, especially if they're beginning to cause you pain. And as we get older, we become more susceptible to wear and tear, and arthritis.

Stretching our hips helps increase our range of motion and relieve pain in our hips. Try these:

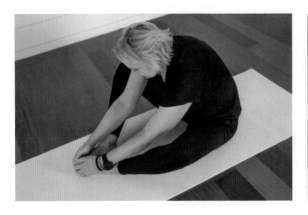

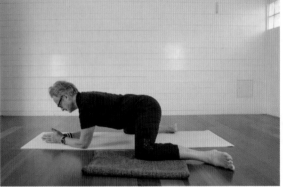

Pose 1: BUTTERFLY

Three minutes
Everyone should do this pose every day. In just three minutes (more if you have time), you'll open your hips and your inner thighs, and feel a lot less stiff.

Pose 2: FROG POSE

Three minutes
Remember to try to fold your feet outward in Frog pose. And don't try to put too much stress on your hips at once. Let your edge, and gravity, do its work.

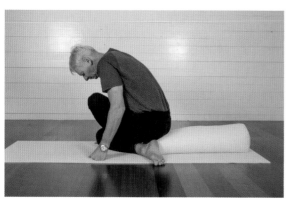

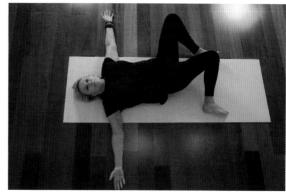

Pose 3: SHOELACE POSE

Three minutes each side

If you have problems doing Shoelace you're not alone. But give it a try as it's an excellent hip opener. Sit on a block, cushion, or bolster and do a Half Shoelace if you can't complete the full pose.

Pose 4: WINDOW WIPERS

As long as you like

A lovely active stretch for your hips as well as the inner and outer muscles of your legs. This is another exercise that's great to do every day. If, of course, you have the time.

Why don't you have the time exactly?

A FIFTEEN-MINUTE FIX TO
shake off sadness

Practitioners of TCM will tell you that if you're feeling down, then maybe your Stomach and Spleen meridians are blocked.

The Stomach meridian starts under your eye and travels to your second toe. The Spleen meridian starts from the outside of your big toe and travels under your armpits.

This fifteen-minute fix helps unblock these lines, hopefully making you feel much happier and balanced.

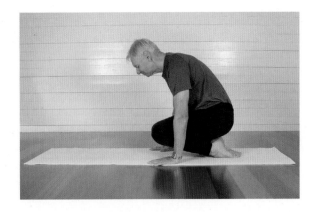

Pose 1: ANKLE STRETCH

One minute or as long as you can
This is a nice way to stimulate your ankles, unblocking the meridians at source. If this pose feels too deep, do Child's pose instead.

Try Dangling for a minute or so as a counterpose.

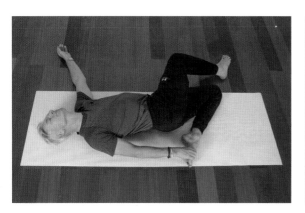

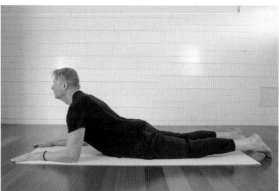

Pose 2: CAT PULLING ITS TAIL

Two to three minutes each side
A really nice stretch to open up your quads and inner thighs. Hug your knees for a minute or so after each pose. You can almost feel the happiness beginning to flow.

Pose 3: SPHINX/SEAL

Three minutes
This pose makes you feel happier and more relaxed and puts back that natural curve to your spine. How happy isn't that?

A FIFTEEN-MINUTE FIX TO
help you mentally declutter

This quick session is more about looking inward than pushing outward. Try thinking from a "me" perspective instead of "them" perspective. It's only when we feel better in ourselves that we can help our family and our friends to be better.

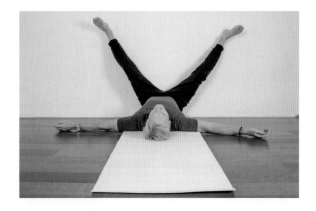

Pose 1: WALL STRADDLE

Five minutes

The easy way into this pose is to lie down parallel to the wall then slide your bottom around as you lift your legs. Once you're there, concentrate on 4x4 breathing. Four seconds in through your nose, hold for four seconds, then four seconds out through your mouth.

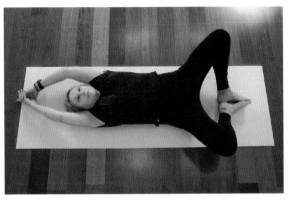

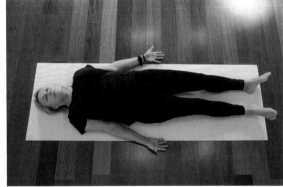

Pose 2: RECLINING BUTTERFLY

Five minutes
If you can, stretch your hands above your head. Maybe lie on a bolster? Concentrate on your breathing.

Have you ever thought much about food and how it can affect your mood? Which foods are good for you? Which ones should you eat more of? And what you should eat/drink less of?

Pose 3: SAVASANA

Five minutes or more
Stay in this relaxing pose for as long as you like. While you're here, scan through your body. How does each part feel? What sensations or thoughts go through your mind as you lie there?

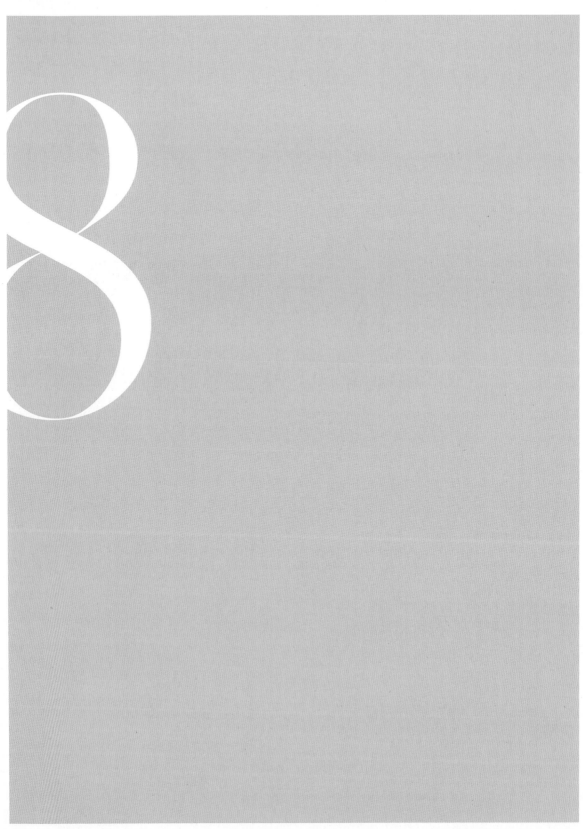

Life hacks
TO ADD TO YOUR YIN

If you're reading this book – and you've read this far – then you know that exercise of any kind is our way to a better quality of life, and in all probability a much longer life.

Exercise keeps us fitter and healthier and can help ward off negative experiences such as poor sleep and depression.

What I've found to be the best with yin yoga are the three major effects of feeling:

Stronger,

More flexible,

Less stressed.

A couple of other small life hacks that I find make big differences are:

TRAIN WITH WEIGHTS

What 50+ fitness gym type are you? The one that never stopped? The one that has lapses? The one who never went? Whichever type you are, we all know that strength training keeps us stronger and helps build muscle mass. That helps preserve our bone density and reduces the risk of diseases such as osteoporosis, heart disease, and arthritis.

Like yin yoga, gym training can improve sleep and reduce depression. So maybe it's time to step up, restart, or go for the first time?

VISIT A PERSONAL TRAINER

Like all types of exercise, if you haven't lifted weights for a long time, see a doctor to make sure you're safe. The next person you should visit is a certified personal trainer who can design a program specially for you.

CONCENTRATE ON YOUR BALANCE

As we age our muscles and nerves become less flexible and our reaction time decreases. This affects our balance, which we need to work on.

Yin yoga is one part of the answer as it helps with flexibility, but we need to include balancing exercises to prevent us from falling—and to make everyday activities like walking, dancing, and cycling so much easier.

Try standing on one leg at a time to see for how long you can do it. Maybe practice when you're cleaning your teeth? As you become proficient, do it again, but this time close your eyes. How did that go?

GO MEDITERRANEAN —WITHOUT GOING TO THE MEDITERRANEAN

We've all read about the Mediterranean diet, so maybe we should adopt it? The diet is high in plant-based foods and some amounts of fish, poultry, and dairy products. It's low on red meat. With benefits including weight loss, a healthier heart, diabetes control, better cognitive function, and possibly a longer life, what's not to like?

One big life hack I've done is to go vegetarian, and I've enjoyed the positive effects already, namely eating food with less calories and no animal fat. I've lost around ten kilos since cutting out meat.

'But I can't live without meat' I hear you say. Fine. Try meat-free Mondays. Then add Thursdays. Then maybe Sundays. And you're already on the way to a healthier life. You don't have to go cold turkey!

TIME TO BEGIN YIN?

I hope this book has inspired you to give yin yoga a try. Or if you've practiced before to keep on doing what you're doing, just more often. And in case you need reminding, yin yoga is a low-impact form of exercise that improves flexibility, relieves stress and helps you sleep.

Good night.

YIN YOGA 50+ MODELS

A big thank you to the beautiful people (in more ways than one) who agreed to help with modeling the poses in this book.

Paul STEELE (AUTHOR)

My yoga journey started about ten years ago when I attended yoga classes to try to improve my flexibility. I wasn't a fan as I thought the poses like Sun Salutations, and Warrior were boring and repetitive. Then I damaged my knee, which stopped me doing the sports I loved.

I found the answer to my problem—yin yoga—without knowing it. I liked the stillness and understood the good each pose was doing. After a few months of doing poses every day I realized that my knee pain had gone. I have full range of motion and enjoy a pain-free active life.

That inspired me to attend a Yoga Alliance 50 teachers' course in Spain a couple of years ago that taught me the practices and principles of yin yoga that I want to share in this book.

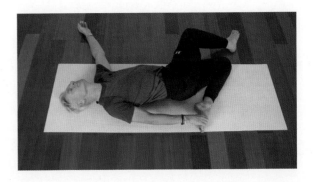

Torgny VIKBLADH

When I was 45, I had constant back problems and lived a very stressful life. I discovered to my horror that my shoulders were so stiff that I could barely put my hands behind my back let alone stretch my arms straight toward the ceiling.

Because of stress and too much sitting, my hip flexors were so tight I had sciatica and pain in my back, neck, and shoulders. Even though I did a little bit of exercise, I was becoming stiffer and stiffer and in more pain. Yoga quickly relieved problems in my back and increased my mobility.

I've run a yoga studio in south Sweden since 2005 and have an RYT 500 Yoga Alliance certification. I've trained thousands of people on various courses over the years.

Tom JOHNSON

I always felt curious about yoga but never did anything about it. Instead I kept jogging, playing tennis, and working out at the gym. I was in good shape but stiff, and with constant minor pains in my back and shoulders. Some years ago I had a partial hip replacement due to osteoarthritis and decided to try yoga to recover.

This felt like a miracle for my body. My hip recovered and as my flexibility increased, the pain in my back and shoulders diminished. And as an extra benefit, yoga helped me to reduce stress and regain good balance, something that has really improved my skiing.

Today I practice yoga four to five times a week, sometimes only for fifteen minutes, but that's enough to make a huge difference to me.

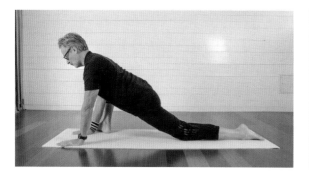
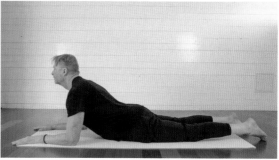

Pia HELLBERG LANNERHEIM

I have always enjoyed all sorts of sports like golf, skiing, and training. Until I got cancer.

After some awful treatment, which seems to have killed off the disease for now, it was time for cancer rehab. What I noticed was that several of the rehab exercises I was given are similar to yin yoga poses. These included Butterfly, Caterpillar, and others specially designed to counteract the effects of radiotherapy.

Being used to yin yoga meant that it was easier for me to adapt the rehab training and probably push on faster than normal.

Additionally, yin yoga helps me sleep better, ease physical and mental tension, and helps me with pain relief.

Karin NILSSON-BRANDENBERGER

Yoga has helped me both physically and mentally. I felt some pain in my right knee when I was skiing or jogging before. Since I started yoga, the pain has vanished and my lower back is also much better. Yoga has helped me feel more grounded and provides me with that "me time" and "time to breath" even when life gets more stressful. It definitely helps me with mindfulness.

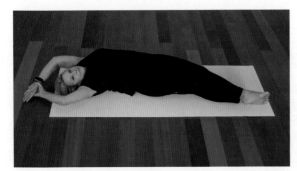

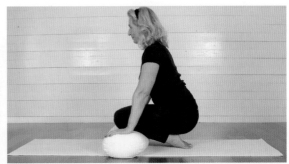

ACKNOWLEDGEMENTS

This book would never have been written without knee pain. So in a masochistic way I have to thank the fact that I was looking round to find ways to alleviate that pain, which I found through yin yoga.

It wouldn't have been possible either without attending a yin yoga teacher's course in Malaga, Spain, led by two outstanding trainers, Ilse-Marie Sobering from House of InnerPower (www.innerpowerhouse.com) and Jane Bakx from Jane Bakx Yoga (www.janebakxyoga.com). Ilse-Marie showed us the beauty of the spiritual side of yin, Jane took us on a deep-dive into the physical and skeletal benefits of a yin yoga practice.

Huge thanks to my partner, Pia Hellberg Lannerheim, who stayed patient as I poured hours of time into researching and writing this book, as well as offering tips and hints on how to make it better.

Kim Malmström, a copywriter colleague, gave up lots of time for little reward in offering ideas on how to improve not just the readability of the texts, but to make them warmer.

Just like cars, this book would be nothing without "old models" who have real stories to tell about how yoga and particularly yin yoga has improved their lives. Thanks to Karin, Pia, Tom, and Torgny.

Thanks for great scientific input Angelica Brandelius and Anders Glemme, and thanks too to Christoffer Wahlgren, Senior Teaching Professional at Wahlgren Golf for verifying the yin for golfers' section.

Sanni Sorma. Without your genius photographic skills and art direction, this book would never have happened.

And thanks to Jon at Lotus Publishing who sees this as a project that is worth sharing.

Thanks guys.